Slow Love
A Polynesian Pillow Book

by
James N. Powell

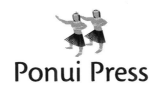

Ponui Press

ISBN 978-0-9800297-0-3
First published in 2008 by
Ponui Press, PO Box 91816, Santa Barbara, CA 93190-1816

To order additional copies, please contact:
Booksurge Publishing
1-886-308-6235
www.booksurge.com
orders@booksurge.com

Cover Design: Jim Powell
Book Design: Renée Michaels Design
Cover Illustration: Daniela Schütt Pozzo
Chapter Heads Art: ©2008 Caren Loebel-Fried
Interior Art: Paul Gauguin

An Important Note

This book was written only to introduce the ancient sexual teachings of the various cultures, as a gesture of goodwill. Because certain exercises, special techniques and teachings that are introduced may be new to certain societies, and because human beings are complicated and delicate in constitution, and because every individual is different, please consult your physician before you try any of the contents of this book, for your own protection, especially if you are suffering from any disease of the sexual organs.

The author and publisher specifically disclaim liability for any loss or risk incurred by the use or application of any of the contents of this book.

Acknowledgements

This book could not have come to light in its present form without the patience and help of Yasuo Yamada, Kana Yamazaki and Renée Michaels.

Ponui, in the native language of Tahiti, means "the immense night." Although *Po* is darkness and night, this darkness is not evil, but good and nurturing, as are the earth and the womb. *Po* is the creative world of night, the magical, immense and dark womb from where our dreaming, our lovemaking, and our visions of spirits blossom forth.

In Europe men and women have sex because they love each other. In the South Seas, they love each other because they have sex.
 – Paul Gauguin

Within the bed curtains,
a guy who can hear his lover's hairpins drop
and not get ideas,
is either very stupid or very wise.
 – from the "Love" section of
 Barbs and Bristles From
 An Archaeophile's Study
 by Lu Zhaoheng (Ming Dynasty)

for Maruata

Contents

Preface 1

Notes from Bed 7

Tokyo in Heat 13

Recumbent Travels 21

On Being Naked 33

On Doing Nothing 61

On Touching 77

The Secret Valley 111

The Silence of the Hummingbird 119

Weaving Together 139

Polynesian Passion–Your Experience 149

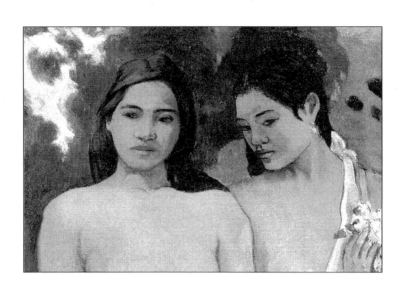

Preface

*D*uring idle spells, when I have had nothing in particular to do, I have jotted down a few lines of this book. In doing so, I have attempted to avoid sounding like a buttoned-down schoolmaster instructing his pupils. For even though I have earned advanced degrees in English literature and the study of tribal religions, I feel my formal education has exercised only a surface influence on my true self. So I have chosen to write in a more casual mode, one that from time to time flows directly from my heart and exposes my reflections and feelings in a way—hopefully—that disarms you, my readers, and establishes a relationship more of friendship. Only in such a comfortable atmosphere, thinking together and at leisure, the kind of ease that allows deepened awareness and mutual trust, can we contemplate with a keen natural sensitivity one of our most natural human acts. Only then can we mutually begin to explore the movement of desire within ourselves and discover its relationship to our capacity for desirelessness.

If my writing helps you discover something deeper and more vital about yourself, it has succeeded. The aboriginal South Sea islanders taught that after joining together with your lover for a long evening, the spirits of the ancestors would gather around to enjoy the deep serenity of the union. Perhaps, while enjoying the teachings in this book, you will feel a group of ancient islanders descending down from the hills of their volcanic isle and gazing long and intently at you, as if wondering if you and your lover are human beings, ghosts, demons or gods.

I was raised on a ranch-farm in Colorado. There I learned about the magical fertility of the soil and about the power and mystery of animals. Growing up far out in the countryside—miles from the nearest town—I found myself in the fading sunset of a still wild, bucolic, red-flannelled, jackleg America of fistfights, cussing and bragging, of home-made ice cream and pie, of quilting bees, of gutbucket bands, of sitting on a porch sipping sarsaparilla, an America nurturing a belief that in wildness and wilderness are lessons that cannot be got from book learning—a backwoods, homespun, boundless place where lanky schoolgirls walked to one-room schoolhouses wearing sunbonnets and calico dresses, or—if they were tomboys, rode a pony—where the woods were sweet with berries, where peaches cost half a buck a bushel, where on a hot day, after forking over two bits at a roadside stand, you would hear the crack of an icy watermelon split open, and where, waiting just beyond a bend in the muddy river, every boy imagined Huck and Jim drifting lazily along on their raft, toes and a fishing line dangling in the cool current…

The ranch-farm was far up a dirt road from a one-intersection town, and so the prevailing reality was one of a vast, undeniable and immaculate silence. In that silence, which had no fence around it, visions and the imagination could blossom forth unimpeded.

I thus learned the immense power of solitude.

On my mother's side of the family we are largely Cherokee. So, from an early age I developed a curiosity about tribal peoples and other cultures, about the most archaic and mythic values on earth, especially if they included the integration of inner silence with activity. And so it was that in my early twenties I developed a keen interest in meditation.

As a young man in his twenties, I also had, naturally, an interest in young women. However, my two fields of interest resulted in something of a conflict. After all, in spiritual and meditation circles, sexual love is often looked down upon. Strict celibacy, or *brahmacharya*, is one of the fundamental cornerstones for serious yogis and yoginis. Spiritual-emotional development, the development of the heart, according to these teachings, is a completely pure realm of life, and can never be integrated with sexual expression. But I observed that even great spiritual leaders are humans first and spiritual leaders second. Why then, I asked myself, repress one's God-given human yearnings? After all, as Sigmund Freud warned us, whatever natural urges we repress will return—often in a stronger and disfigured form. There must be some way—I thought—that one's sexual and spiritual-emotional life can be integrated gently, in a way that they nourish each other. If a man can love Spirit, then why can he not love a woman? Why cannot spiritual experience and human love enhance each other? Why not explore love between a man and woman as a kind of meditation?

Because I was thinking in this direction, it was natural that I would discover the Chinese Taoist and Indian Tantra teachings on sexual yoga, which I explored. Yet, they seemed based on control, and what I was looking for was a way of integrating human and spiritual love in a most natural and gentle manner. Luckily, in the mountains near my home at that time lived a Tahitian woman. She became my friend and invited me to a dinner party at her house. Being something of a bookworm, after dinner I found myself thumbing through the many volumes on her bookshelves—especially one on some wonderful teachings of South Seas sexual ways. Here, finally, I had found a completely natural way to integrate emotional and spiritual development with sexual union. It is these teachings that I focus on in this volume, with some asides to Taoist and Tantric wisdom.

I use the term "Polynesia" in the original sense, which included all of Oceania—Melanesia and Micronesia as well as what is today known as Polynesia. Those readers who wish to delve deeply into more academic studies of South Pacific life might wish to begin with one of the following: *South Sea Maidens: Western Fantasy and Sexual Politics in the South Pacific* (Michael Sturma); "First Contacts" in Polynesia, the Samoan Case (1722–1848): Western Misunderstandings about Sexuality and Divinity. *Pacific Affairs*, 79 (Dan Taulapapa McMullin); European Intimidation and the Myth of Tahiti. *Journal of Pacific History*, 4 (W. H. Pearson); Possessing Tahiti. *Archeology in Oceania*, 21 (Greg Dening); *European Imagery and Colonial History in the Pacific* (Toon van Meijl & Paul van der Grijp, Eds.); *Tahitians: Mind and Experience in the Society Islands* (Robert I. Levy); *Two Tahitian Villages: A Study in Comparison* (Douglas Oliver); *Coming of Age in Samoa* (Margaret Mead); *Love in the South Seas: Sex and Family Life of the Polynesians, Based on Early Accounts as Well as Observations by the Noted Swedish Anthropologist* (Bengt Danielsson); and *Marquesan Sexual Behavior: An Anthropological Study of Polynesian Practices* (Robert C. Suggs).

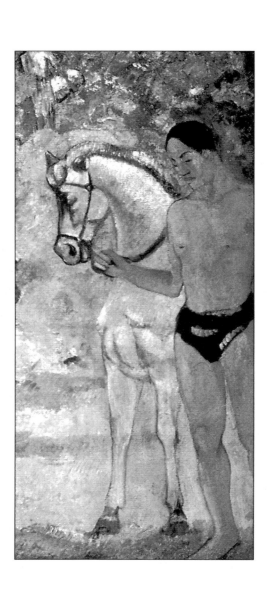

Notes From Bed

*I*n he realm of passion one does not have to seek far and wide to find know-it-alls. For thousands of years the world has been full of wise-guys, playboys, pillow books, pornographic encyclopedias, sexological treatises by overeducated doctors, and the blabberings of love gurus from every continent. However, what does the world have to show for all such sagacity but a swelling and sweaty mass of reeking bodies that—for a few minutes—feverishly claw at each other like cats and pant like dogs?

Usually the idle hours of new lovers are devoted to such passion. Yet, the flame soon fades. The honeymoon is soon over. Too many relationships fall apart. Marriages end in divorce or in sexless boredom.

This book will demonstrate how the clawing and clutching style of passion that most couples engage in is actually at fault in ending many relationships. As science informs us—the brain chemistry produced by conventional sexual relations is more likely to drive people apart than to keep them happily together, because it annihilates the brain chemicals associated with feelings of being in love.

However, some of the aboriginal South Sea islanders enjoyed a style of slow, languid lovemaking that actually increases the level of brain chemicals involved with feelings of being in love.

And, when you think about it, if you have ever experienced an episode of lovemaking that took you utterly beyond this world—that had a lotus-like aroma, that with the first long embrace moistened your lips and throat, that with the second embrace broke the deep loneliness of your heart, that with the third raised a slight perspiration, that with the fourth found all the wrongs of life passing away through your pores, that with the fifth left you weightless and with the sixth transported both your lover and yourself up to the realms of the immortals—it was a kind of lazy lovemaking, a lovemaking in which your lover and you lolled around languidly in each other's arms for hours, simply luxuriating in the life of the body: its rhythms, its enjoyments—its capacity for play and a lasting sense of peace that is sacred.

In the South Seas of long ago, on tranquil mornings when honeyed sunlight spilled through the palms, painting the bodies of lovers in stripes of light and shadow, while millions of other couples in Europe and Asia were going at it as busily as beavers or penning encyclopedias of fleshly sins, South Seas lovers pushed to the utter limit the time they spent just loafing idle and unmotivated in each other's embrace, bodies in serene contact, resting slothfully, going absolutely nowhere, feeling their cares evaporate, hearing their hearts beat in indolent harmony, perhaps listening to the song of a bird, or idly watching shadows of hibiscus flowers dance across the wall, perhaps dozing off in a sweet reverie, thus becoming lords of their rustic South Seas huts, which began to glow like palaces of joy as the frenzies of the civilized world, unknown to them, slipped by unnoticed.

Deep in their silent embraces, at times all breath would cease. They would tremble within a calm silence, their hearts sensitive to the smallest of things and the most subtle of feelings: soft breezes ruffling the surface of the lagoon, the faint rustle of trade winds in palm fronds. In utter equipoise, their hearts were devoted to undivided absorption, a moment perfectly beyond time, with no colors to disturb an inner glowing, not a sound to mar heartfelt stillness and not a word to break the unity.

Blessed with the aroma of countless such unions, why did no South Seas sexual slowpokes pen a volume about the spiritual satisfaction found in sensual sluggishness? The answer is apparent. Even if they had had a system of writing, they would have been immediately confronted with a monstrous paradox. If it was true that they were really supreme sexual slackers, they would certainly be too slothful to obey any wandering notion that they should write a book, to muster up all the effort it takes to descend from a timeless embrace, to untangle one's limbs from those of one's beloved, to drag one's body out of bed, to unsheathe a pen, to dip the quill in dark ink, to prop one's spine against the back of a chair, to sit before a writing table with a kettle of tea steaming noisily (which one would have had to put on the fire) and to scribble even a few half-coherent words.

If these South Seas lovers had, miraculously, accomplished even a few lines, any intelligent and truly languorous reader would certainly have concluded that they were not at all worthy authorities on the art of laziness, and would probably have already given up reading. After all—the reader will have concluded—a truly unmotivated master of sensual indolence would simply forgo all conventional forms of writing. The only ode he would know would be the one inscribed by his writhing lover's eyelashes scribbling their trembling calligraphy upon his neck. And if this master of languid loving were to worship a god, his deity would surely satisfy his own sexual passions simply by digging a hole in the ground, inserting his penis, and waiting for an earthquake.

Further, truly indolent readers may wonder how one could possibly explore the spiritual subtleties of female sexual response enough to write an art of erotics if one were busying oneself taking notes on every swelling of flesh and sigh of surrender. As Lin Yutang, a renowned Chinese master of idleness once wrote, the Chinese failed to develop a science of zoology simply because "a Chinese scholar cannot stare at a fish without immediately thinking of how it tastes in the mouth."

Since we have neither a written *ars erotica* penned by passionate and unashamed ancient South Sea islanders nor any odes to physical love from their mostly Christian descendents, I, although a reasonably lazy fellow, have taken up the task of writing one, drawing upon various anthropological and anecdotal accounts as well as personal experiences. I would like to suggest in my defense (for a lazy man does not argue), that it has taken me many years to jot down even these few sleepy phrases and that it is perhaps better to read a ninety-seven-percent authority on lazy love than no authority at all.

In fact, I would like to suggest that once having read this book, you, my readers, will have learned to become sufficiently slothful to be able to shun all teachings on matters of sex, to throw into the flames all pillow books, polls and pronouncements of love pundits— including this one. You will have learned by reading this book to become educated in such matters solely within the sensual and absolutely authoritative embrace of your lover and the glow between your two hearts.

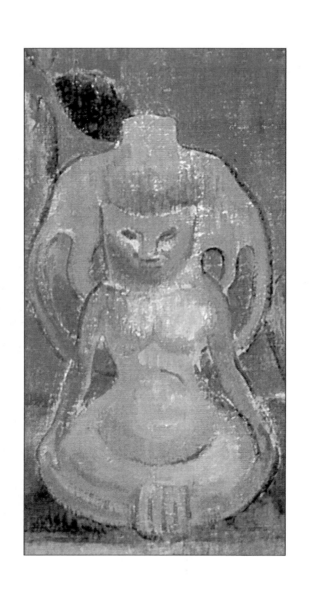

Tokyo In Heat

A revolution is taking place in Japan. And as history has proven, revolutions cannot be evaded and they seldom go backward. As yet, it is a small revolution, and its heat is felt not in bloody battles on the streets, but in the hearts and bodies of lovers in private recesses of their own bedrooms.

The revolution I write of is a quiet revolution, a lazy revolution, and a recumbent one, because it is a revolution of languid, laidback loving. Thousands of couples in Japan have discovered that when embracing—at the pivot between stimulation and stillness, at the conjunction between stirring and repose—dwells something mysterious, luminous. To relax into that light, to become absorbed in it, is to become free of the floods of images that normally busy the mind, and to join souls with one's lover.

This sexual revolution began a few years ago with the release of the Japanese translation of my book *Energy and Eros*, an exploration of sexuality in various cultures, including Polynesia. At first, only a modest number of volumes sold, but couples who explored the Polynesian lovemaking teachings detailed in the last chapter found themselves becoming more relaxed about lovemaking, and subsequently enjoying deeper and more fulfilling levels of intimacy. Moreover, they began to find that the fullness they felt as the result of

Polynesian passion overflowed into their everyday lives. They discovered that South Seas sensuality was not only about sex, but also about the heart and relationship. And, sitting in coffee houses, women who discovered the deliciousness of loving lazily began telling their girlfriends about it.

One of the book's early admirers was the great Japanese writer Hiroyuki Itsuki. Impressed with its unique teachings on the art of love, in 2002 he penned two volumes—*Silent Love* and *Twelve Chapters on Love*—introducing my thoughts on what had become known in Japan as "Polynesian sex" to a wider Japanese audience.

This caused a stir in the Tokyo media, and Japanese Internet chat was soon buzzing with discussions of "Polynesian sex." The *Weekly Gendai*, Japan's premier men's magazine, ran a twelve-week series on modern lovemaking. The aim of the series was to restrain men from their sprint to orgasm, urging them to love in a slower, more sensual, more pacific fashion. One article lauded languid, laidback Polynesian lovemaking, during which lovers stroke and caress each other's bodies for a least an hour before penetration. "A lot of Japanese men have the idea the best sex you can have is fast, macho, American-style sex," said Kazuo Takahashi, editor of the magazine.

Women's magazines also picked up on the slow-love trend, with *Nikkei Woman*'s 2005 sex issue recommending the Polynesian approach as an antidote to the "too-hard, too-fast" loving that seems all too common. Soon after that, pop music star Masaharu Fukuyama, appearing on All Night Nippon, recommended Polynesian lovemaking to his many thousands of fans.

As a result of the media exposure, a lot of Japanese women suddenly found themselves desirous of making love at a Polynesian pace, and—in order to meet the sudden demand—more than a few Japanese playboys feigned expertise in South Seas sensuality.

As I pen these lines, thousands of Japanese web sites mention Polynesian sex and it has become a topic of Internet blogs. In this way, Polynesian passion is slowly and lazily changing sensuality on the isles that gave the world *shunga* (erotic paintings found in Japanese "bride's books") and *manga* (Japanese comics).

What types of experiences do couples report? Both men and women seem to be benefiting. For some, South Seas sensuality simply makes conventional lovemaking—including orgasm—better.

MEN

- When in a deep embrace, I feel our love spreading quietly from the silence in my heart. It is as if the boundaries of our bodies dissolve, as if we become like clouds, and then like rain upon the earth. In being these, we lose ourselves in these.
- I feel so much more emotionally intimate with my girl, because I am more aware of her very subtle responses—not just her physical ones—and I feel them much more directly.
- I experience an unearthly pleasure vibrating in me from head to toe. I have never felt such a sensation making love in the conventional thrusting manner.
- I felt vivid pleasure, even more intense than the first time I made love as a teenager.
- I think I felt how a woman feels when she comes to ecstasy in love.
- I used to wonder, anxiously, if my sweetheart actually felt fulfillment in my embrace, but now I no longer wonder.

WOMEN

- I came for the first time, but what I enjoy most is our quiet sessions, because the quietness and the tenderness of our love flow into our lives long after we stop embracing.
- Before I experienced pain during lovemaking. Now I experience pleasure.
- My skin is covered with love dew, and I flow with love juice, for the first time.
- Once I begin feeling waves of fulfillment, I remain in that space, and continue—like flying!
- I enjoy it a lot when we are still, and our skin is simply touching, for a long while.
- As we near the end, my body becomes so responsive and sensitive to feather-light caresses.

As you can see from these experiences, lovers who have enjoyed Polynesian sex are beginning to dive into the deep and tranquil ocean of the heart, and their relationships are overflowing with peace and feelings of unity.

Our sexual nature, after all, is not separate from the vast universe of Nature that surrounds us, and I think almost everyone has gone for a hike in the mountains. Maybe you start out in the morning, when the dew is still on the flowers. As you hike, you enjoy the views that unfold before your eyes. Perhaps you see a butterfly, a bird or a deer. But when they notice you, they run for cover. As the Greek philosopher Heraclites put it—Nature likes to hide. And, as you are hiking, you will notice that Nature does hide as it hears you coming.

Around noon you will probably feel hungry. You find some shade under a tree, unpack your lunch and dig in. After eating, you sit back against the trunk of the tree just to relax and enjoy a little leisure before you move on.

The first thing you may notice is the silence. You have been hiking all morning, but your heavy breathing, the rhythmic sound of your boots on the trail and thoughts of your destination have not let you relish the delicious depth of silence you now suddenly realize has been there all the while.

Then, in this silence, other treasures begin to unfold themselves before your eyes. After all, you are sitting against a tree, and you blend in with the natural environment. Now, if a deer wanders by, the creature may not even notice you, unless you move, even if the deer is quite close. Or, a bird might land almost at your feet, or a snake might come slithering by or a butterfly settle on your nose.

You may suddenly notice for the first time the feel of the earth beneath you, the blended fragrances of the forest, the muted roar of a distant waterfall, the notes of many bird songs.

In short—you will notice that Nature, which likes to hide, seems to be gradually unveiling her mysteries before your very eyes. The longer you sit, the more Nature lifts her veils. And what have you done to enjoy this beautiful awareness of the natural world that surrounds you?

Nothing. You have simply become more lazy.

Nature has not changed. You have simply become more quiet, and are thus able to enjoy her more fully.

You, as a human being, are part of Nature, also. And in this book you will be exploring your sexual-emotional nature. You will discover that—just as you see more of Nature when you are quiet—you enjoy more of your own sexual-emotional nature when you allow yourself to become more still—more aware.

In order to discover more quiet inside yourself, you are going to explore some very simple, fundamental things: the way you breathe, the way you touch your lover and the way you think and feel about him or her.

In these explorations you are not seeking a "correct" breathing or touching or feeling. You are quite simply exploring and discovering the nature of breathing, touching and feeling—by becoming more quiet.

What is really happening when you touch your lover? Are you performing? Are you trying to stimulate your lover in order to create an orgasm? Have you ever touched your lover in a way that has no goal in mind? Have you ever sat in a warm bath with your lover and, not attempting to seduce or stimulate, washed your lover's face tenderly, in order to really sense the expressions that form on your lover's lips, in your lover's eyes—in order to really see who is really there?

The sighs of your lover, the smile or cloud of sadness that momentarily shadows the face, the boldness or reticence of the gaze, all can be overlooked if you are merely attempting to seduce, and all these subtle physical indications help you to know not just the outer appearance, but also the inner energy, the affections, the spirit of your lover. All of these use little to comprehend much, like the single blossom that lets you know Spring is coming, which helps you to feel the tone of the coming season.

Thus, as a lover, you are not a mere observer, but a creature who, sensitive to the tone of your beloved, is able to share in it as a path that leads you to your lover's heart.

Such "study" has no end, and you are your own authority in this—once you learn to become quiet.

This book is an invitation to re-examine the way you touch,

breathe, feel and make love. It is an invitation to discover what is really authentic in your loving and what is there just from your cultural and psychological conditioning, your habit and the patterns of your addictions.

Yet, the explorations in this book are not only mental. You will be exploring and discovering with your heart, your relationships, your breath, your fingers, your entire body—a more sensitive way of relating to your lover.

You will consider in much more depth the cultural, emotional, relational, and physical areas you must contemplate in order to live a truly nourishing and regenerative sexuality. You will let your own, spontaneous lust and love become your koan.

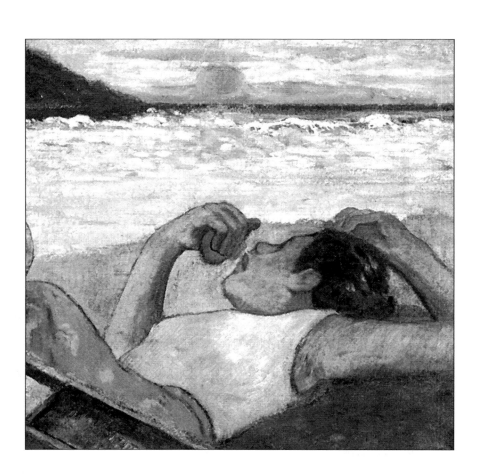

Recumbent Travels

*I*n a sunny village in Southern Italy once lived a fellow who was a great professor of laziness. Yet, unlike other professors, this professor had nothing to profess. His entire teaching consisted of saying nothing and doing nothing. Understandably, he had attracted no disciples. He lived in a rather dilapidated villa he had inherited, and in the golden afternoon light of late summer, as the grapes fattened in the vineyards of the surrounding hills, he could be found stretched out in a hammock in the dappled shade of his fig orchard.

Now, by this season all his neighbors' figs had been industriously harvested, packed, labeled, shipped to market, haggled over, and brought home by busy moms to adorn tables and sweeten mouths between meals or to accompany cheese and wine after dinners. But the figs of the great professor of laziness, still hanging by their slender stems, by this time had swollen to such sweetness that they were not shippable; the skins had begun to develop vertical cracks and the syrup to ooze out the bottoms.

In a village to the south of the great professor lived a man who had a famously lazy teenage son. In fact, so sluggish was the teen that the father had given up all but one hope: He had heard of the professor of laziness, and decided that if his son could be good for nothing else, he could learn from the professor some hidden subtleties about the spiritual dimensions of laziness, and at least achieve something in that, much neglected, field of human endeavor.

So, he put his son on a donkey and led the beast over the hills, through the vineyards, and over the streams leading to the village where lived the great professor of laziness.

When they arrived at the village, after a journey of some days, the father made inquiries and was directed to the professor's villa, which was surrounded by a high wall interrupted only by a rude, broken gate. The father, with his son behind him, knocked on the gate, but received no reply.

Over the top of the gate the father could see the tops of the fig trees, laden with overripe fruit, and peering through a broken board, could see just the bare foot of the professor, with a few flies circling his big toe. Carefully the father opened the gate and entered, with his son dragging along behind him. There in the middle of the fig orchard they beheld the professor of laziness stretched out on his back like a sleeping dog, dozing tranquilly in his hammock. The father was overjoyed, walked over to the professor and took a seat. Meanwhile the son found another hammock, and availing himself of it, soon was dozing peacefully in the shade.

The father introduced himself to the professor of laziness, but the learned man said nothing and did nothing. Even if a fly would land on his face, he would not notice, but simply go on snoring. However, suddenly a fig dropped from the branches above the professor; the professor's arm shot suddenly out with the speed of a lizard's tongue, his cupped hand forming a perfect cradle for the soft belly of the fig as it fell. Having caught the fig, the professor brought it to his mouth, sucked out the sweet syrup and seeds, and spat out the skin, which fell to a pile of fig skins that littered the ground.

At this sign of movement, the father took the opportunity to address the professor again. The professor condescended to open one eye enough to blurrily regard the father. The father said that he was much impressed with the demonstration of laziness he had just witnessed—and begged the professor to accept his son as a student.

At that moment, however, another fig, overcome by the weight of its own sweet syrup, dropped from the branches above the lazy son. In fact, the fig fell through the air straight toward the mouth of the lazy son, where it landed on his teeth, automatically disemboweling its own soft belly, which spewed its syrupy continents onto the tongue of the boy, whose hands remained folded peacefully across his chest as he dozed.

The great professor of laziness, upon beholding this, sat bolt upright. He opened both eyes wide, and he opened his mouth. "Sir!" he proclaimed to the father, "Your son is a greater master of laziness than I. I have nothing to teach him. Quite to the contrary, I must learn from him."

The lazy son, however, continued dreaming, unimpressed with the praise of the great professor of laziness. He continued dozing, interrupted only by the falling of an occasional fig, which somehow managed to offer its contents to his tongue in the same manner as had the first.

As a teenage boy I was, of course, hungry for a mouthful of the opposite sex, but too lazy to pursue the prey in her natural habitat. Why chase girls, I reasoned, if I could simply lie in bed and conjure them up mentally? Thus, often, I would find myself lazing about in bed dreaming of islands.

23

The islands I dreamed of were not just any islands, because I did not want just any girl. They had to be islands of the South Pacific—islands of grass huts and blue lagoons and surf whitening on distant reefs. And, in my listless mind I would block everything out and would paint a mental picture of a Polynesian sunset: A family gathered in a cookhouse, enjoying mounds of poi, bananas and fish of every color. After dinner, there is not much conversation. A cool breeze stirs the palm fronds, everyone cleans up, and around the silent house the darkening evening is disturbed only by the distant thunder of waves or the occasional bark of a dog. Mats and bedding are brought out, lamps snuffed, and sleep comes.

Yet, nightfall does not bring sleep to everyone, for at dinner the young men are freshly bathed. They wear only a piece of cloth, wrapped around the waist. They have flashlights and guitars ready. The young women, as well, have just emerged from a stream or a pool beneath a waterfall, their bodies fragrant and aglow with coconut oil scented with sandalwood. Behind their ears they wear a hibiscus. And so, as most on the island succumb to dreams, the young men slip off into the darkness, and the young women lie awake on their sleeping mats, feigning slumber until their parents fall asleep.

And so I would lie in bed, my mind resting in silence, imagining what pleasures await those young Polynesians in the deep and fragrant folds of the black tropic night.

Deep within my pubescent psyche—as in the psyches of many American teens of the period—beckoned an image so sensual that I could come close to it only in fantasy or dream.

The setting, as I have already indicated, is important. It could be any of thousands of mere specks of sand lost somewhere within the vast blue, balmy latitudes of the South Pacific. I could imagine myself arriving at such an island neither on a passenger plane nor aboard a cruise ship. That would be too direct, and require too much effort. Because I was so lazy, reaching the South Pacific isle could not be an act of my own will. It was necessary that I be carried there by something greater than myself—by a force to which I could only surrender. It was necessary that I be washed ashore—marooned in the style of the great beachcombers of yore.

The bays of the island would be ringed by a dark line of palms swaying along their curves, gray trunks swelling gently outward over a placid lagoon. The trees would crowd the beach, fringing it and climbing steep slopes that rise beyond the narrow littoral. Beyond, I would see towering tiers of dark, volcanic peaks and rising vales lost in opalescent canopies of clouds, so that I could not determine if the clouds borrowed their hues from the peaks, or the peaks from the clouds.

Washed ashore like a piece of driftwood, I would drag myself into a dappled patch of shade underneath a towering palm, and surrender to the warm, soft sand. There I would fall asleep.

The next morning, as I slept, the roar of the surf on the reef, the smell of thousands of unseen and unknown flowers, and the glare of the sun upon my closed eyes would sift down through my dream within a dream—swimming within the sea of my mind. I would attempt to open my eyes, but my vision would be a little blurry. I would hear a mellifluous giggle. I would rub my eyes in earnest and look up.

And only then would I see her—the taboo presence haunting my dreams: I would see that I was being held in the mischievous gaze of a creature radiant with the ambrosial happiness of youth. Slender, dark, long legged, and dressed only in a hibiscus and a cascade of black hair falling almost to her ankles, she would regard me with a shy but sultry gaze shining from large, melting eyes set below dark brows. These would only accentuate her breasts, which would be the color of dark honey. Her pert nipples and full lips would be black as figs. Yet, she would seem totally unaware of her nakedness. "Aloha" I would venture. At this, she would only throw back her head and laugh, flashing a row of pearly teeth and exposing her throat. Every curve of her body would be smeared with coconut oil scented with sandalwood powder and flowers.

With the musky scent of her body pulling me under its spell, she would lead me to her thatched hut. There, I would spend idle days with her in tranquility—fishing, drinking the juice of coconuts, bathing in soft breezes or hunting for flowers to twine in her hair. At night I would dive naked with her in a placid lagoon, and then, reclining upon moonlit, white coral sands, swim within the warm embrace of her raw sensuality until my passion reached its youthful conclusion. Then I would fall into a deep sleep.

I was not the only teenage boy to succumb to such fantasies. Nor was I even a little original in my imaginings. After all, the image I have just written of has a long history and has remained essentially unchanged since the eighteenth century, when it was created on a balmy morning in 1767.

On that morning the *Dolphin*, a British sailing vessel anchored in the blue waters of Tahiti's Matavai Bay, was greeted by a flotilla of canoes, each ornamented with the seductive figure of a copper-limbed young nymph. The myth that has come down in history from this first encounter of Europeans with Tahitians is that the loose morals of these Tahitian beauties is what made them warmly welcome the sailors. But this is, as you will see in the next chapter, merely a myth. It is a myth, however, that continues to this day.

A year later, in 1768, when the *Boudeuse*, commanded by Louis-Antoine de Bougainville (for whom the bougainvillea flower is named), anchored in the same tropical paradise, a dripping wet Tahitian temptress clamored aboard, flaunting herself nakedly before the eyes of the sailors. This brief enticement no doubt aroused considerable anticipation among the crew, who were not disappointed the next day when they rowed ashore to find a fragrant and fertile land fed by streams and waterfalls, bathed in pure air and filled with voluptuous beauties.

A year after that, Captain James Cook's ship, the *Endeavor*, arrived in Tahiti. The notes left by Cook and the expedition's naturalist, Joseph Banks, illustrated the area's flora and fauna. But real interest in the documents arose only years later, when John Hawkesworth used them to write a summation of the expedition, entitled *Voyages*. This volume included descriptions of naturalist Banks' sexual exploits with Tahitian women as well as accounts of the very natural sexual behavior of the island's populace.

Herman Melville brought the image to American readers in his novel *Typee* (1846), a semi-autobiographical story of a sailor who went native in the Marquesas, after a pod of young native women swam out to meet the ship, danced voluptuously in lantern light before the admiring crew, and then spent the night with them in wild abandon.

The event that transformed the imagination of Europeans was not any factual account of Polynesian pleasures, but publication of a novel written by Julian Viaud, who was re-named Loti by his Tahitian lovers. His novel, *Le marriage de Loti*, published in 1880, seduced a generation of readers with the wisdom of forsaking icy European winters for the tranquility and languor of romantic Tahiti, where Loti wrote of his love with the dark-eyed and serene Rarahu, and of nights with her as all-enveloping as the depths of her long cascades of ebony hair.

South Seas fantasies took on mythic dimensions in the life and works of French painter Paul Gauguin. The artist's friend Émile Bernard, who had read Loti, had given Gauguin a foretaste of the delights he would find in Tahiti. Thus Gauguin fantasized that in the silent beauty of Tahiti's tropical nights, he would be able to listen to the soft murmuring music of his heart in amorous harmony with the mysterious beings around him. Indeed, he did find mysterious beings: Titi, Tehaurana, Pau'ura and Vaeoho are the names of just some of the women the painter took as lovers. Gauguin left the world a splendid array of paintings of calm-eyed Tahitian women, which have lured aspiring beachcombers to far reaches of the Pacific in search of the paradise of Polynesian loveliness he portrayed.

When anthropologist Branislaw Malinowski published *The Sex Life of Savages*—his observations of the sexual mores of inhabitants of the Trobriand Islands, and Margaret Mead quickly followed with her title *Coming of Age in Samoa*—both volumes painting Pacific isles as sexual utopias—it just added more fuel to the fire. Mead's work on the love life of Samoan maidens was the best selling anthropology book ever.

The story that really sealed the image of the Polynesian nymph in the world's popular imagination, however, was the voyage of the H. M. S. *Bounty*. In 1789 the ship had anchored in Tahiti for five months, where the crew had ample time to acquaint themselves with the Tahitian women. Upon departure, taking on a cargo of breadfruit trees and sailing for the West Indies, twenty-five sailors led by Fletcher Christian seized control of the ship. Some of the mutineers stopped by Tahiti to be reunited with their Tahitian lovers, and then made their way to Pitcairn Island, whereas others remained in Tahiti. It seems unthinkable that the actions of so small a group of men in such a remote quarter of the globe could exercise such a vast influence on the popular imagination. Yet, to date five films have been made about the mutiny, with Clark Gable, Errol Flynn, Marlon Brando and Mel Gibson each taking a turn at playing Fletcher Christian. It was the Brando version that I saw when I was coming of age and new seas of hormones were beginning to wash through my blood. The film sparked my interest in the South Seas.

Stories and novels of encounters between early European voyagers and Polynesian damsels provided the template for today's travel brochures of white-sand beaches and the modern sexual fantasies of the South Pacific. It became natural for those reading accounts of the South Seas or seeing films such as *Mutiny on the Bounty* to imagine Tahiti as a paradisiacal garden covered with a vast canopy of blossoming trees of every variety; of lovely natives bathing in the waters of slender cascades that leap down cliffs amidst verdant herbage; of maidens swimming in the waters of a blue lagoon, propelling themselves with the ease and grace of mermaids: gliding along barely beneath the surface, then surfacing, diving again, and darting off at angles, turning on their sides to flaunt the beauty of their forms; of women seated on the green banks of waterfalls, fanning out their hair and rubbing scented oils onto their bodies. Their long, luxuriant and glossy tresses fall over their shoulders to their waists and their sisters sit serenely behind them, plaiting their hair with golden blossoms.

Such are the images of Polynesian sensuality that have become popular all over the world. The image of the Polynesian nymph was not simply added on as one more image in the vast collection of erotic images that have for millennia ignited imaginations. It became a central image, and during some exotica-obsessed decades *the* central image of sensual femininity. At a time when the European imagination was painting tribal peoples worldwide as "noble savages," the Polynesian maiden came to be the longed-for "nubile savage."

However, it is always necessary to ask questions about things that have become central and taken for granted. Thus, regarding the image of the Polynesian nymph, some important questions arise: Were the Tahitian women really as willing as the myth suggests? What if traditional Polynesian sexuality was not based on images? Further, what if traditional Polynesians lived in a culture that was entirely free of pornography or sexual imaginings of any kind? What if mental images of our lover actually stand in the way of deep sexual communion?

If it is true that the aboriginal Polynesian mind was relatively void of sexual images, then we reach a most startling conclusion: The worldwide fascination with the image of the dark, bare-breasted hula girl under the coconut palm can have nothing at all to do with Polynesian passion. And if that is true, then what is the real nature of South Seas sensuality before the arrival of the Europeans? It must have been a union between lovers that transcends all the images—all the advertising and porn that fuel much of the "civilized world's" sex.

All the world's imaginings about Polynesian damsels may be missing the point entirely.

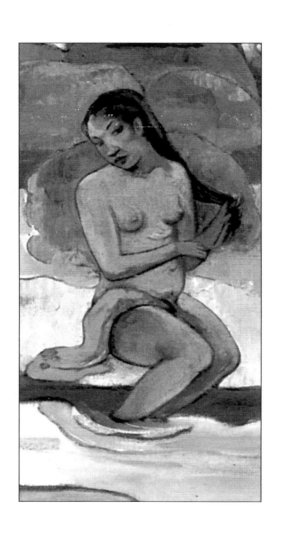

On Being Naked

On his first voyage to Tahiti, as the painter Gauguin was exploring the island, he passed a night in the forest, alone. As he writes in *Noa Noa*,

> On the following day, very early, I took up my way again.
>
> The river became more and more irregular. It was now brook, now torrent, now waterfall. It wound about in a strangely capricious way, and sometimes seemed to flow back into itself. I was continually losing the path, and often had to advance swinging from branch to branch with the hands, scarcely touching the ground.
>
> From the bottom of the water cray-fish of extraordinary shape looked at me as if to say, "What are you doing here?" And hundred-year-old eels fled at my approach.
>
> Suddenly, at an abrupt turn, I saw a naked young woman leaning against a projecting rock. She was caressing it with both hands, rather than using it as a support. She was drinking from a spring which in silence trickled from a great height among the rocks.
>
> After she had finished drinking, she let go of the

rock, caught the water in both hands, and let it run down between her breasts. Then, though I had not made the slightest sound, she lowered her head like a timid antelope which instinctively scents danger and peered toward the thicket where I remained motionless. My look did not meet hers. Scarcely had she seen me, than she plunged below the surface, uttering the word, "*Taëhaë* (furious)."

Quickly I looked into the river—no one, nothing— only an enormous eel, which wound in and out among the small stones at the bottom.

∼

There is a reason why "civilized" people spend time fantasizing about glimpsing—through gaps in the bamboo—a bare Polynesian woman or man, waist deep in water, flower in hair, bathing under a waterfall.

It is because they do not find such scenes on the sidewalks of New York, London, Tokyo and Beijing.

There are, however, two kinds of nakedness: physical and mental. We all know what it means to be physically naked. But mental nakedness is something beyond thought. Mental nakedness requires a truly idle mind, which is rare, because no mind can luxuriate in idleness unless it is free from the spells cast by images. Only such an utterly blank mind—stripped of all images and doing absolutely nothing— can be truly free. For, if there is an image in the mind, the mind is busily engaged with that image.

Most so-called civilized people are naked neither physically nor mentally. They spend a great deal of time selecting the clothing they will wear and then spend even more time either looking at photos, films or drawings of bodies denuded of most attire, or imagining or fantasizing about them. In fact sexual perversities and fetishes are based on images that have become fixed in the mind. It is thus common for sexual deviants to be much more interested in some part of their lover's body than in the actual feelings and life of their lover.

The aboriginal Polynesians, on the other hand, because they lived in a land of eternal summer, did not need to wear much. Although on some occasions they would dress fully and elegantly, frequently, unlike Europeans and most Asians, the Polynesians felt no need to cover most of the body, including women's breasts. And because women's breasts were often physically naked, Polynesian men had no need to form images and fetishes of them in their minds. As writer Camille Paglia has observed, there is nothing less erotic than a nudist colony.

Gauguin, writing long before Paglia, commented in *Noa Noa* that the lack of gender differences and sexual tension in Tahitian society is brought about by the population being accustomed to and comfortable with the unclothed human form:

> Among peoples that go naked, as among animals, the difference between the sexes is less accentuated than in our climates. Thanks to our cinctures and corsets we have succeeded in making an artificial being out of woman. She is an anomaly, and Nature herself, obedient to the laws of heredity, aids us in complicating and enervating her. We carefully keep her in a state of nervous weakness and muscular inferiority, and in guarding her from fatigue, we take away from her possibilities of development. Thus modeled on a bizarre ideal of slen-

derness to which, strangely enough, we continue to adhere, our women have nothing in common with us, and this, perhaps, may not be without grave moral and social disadvantages.

On Tahiti the breezes from forest and sea strengthen the lungs, they broaden the shoulders and hips. Neither men nor women are sheltered from the rays of the sun nor the pebbles of the seashore. Together they engage in the same tasks with the same activity or the same indolence. There is something virile in the women and something feminine in the men.

This similarity of the sexes makes their relations the easier. Their continual state of nakedness has kept their minds free from the dangerous pre-occupation with the "mystery" and from the excessive stress which among civilized people is laid upon the "happy accident" and the clandestine and sadistic colors of love. It has given their manners a natural innocence, a perfect purity. Man and woman are comrades, friends rather than lovers, dwelling together almost without cease, in pain as in pleasure.

However, when European sailors arrived in Tahiti they would stare at the breasts of Tahitian *vahines*. The women really could not understand and would poke fun of the sailors, calling them "peepers." Looking at a beautiful *vahine* on the beach, the European sailors saw a naked woman. Looking at the same *vahine*, Polynesian men saw only a woman. They had no fixation on nudity and therefore harbored no fetishes about parts of women's bodies.

Thus, aboriginal Polynesians went naked not only physically, but also mentally. For like Adam and Eve in the Garden of Eden, they did not have much mental concern about physical nudity until confronted by the voyeuristic European perspective. Before European contact, for Polynesian women to display their breasts in pubic was completely natural—no more startling than showing one's nose. However, the Europeans brought with them "civilization," and it was not long before many Polynesians were as prim, proper, "decently" clothed, sexually uptight and perverse as their European conquerors.

A revealing American film depicting the almost Nazi-like state of sexual repression that descended upon many Polynesian isles is the 1953 classic, *Return to Paradise*. Based on the first story in James Michener's *Tales of the South Pacific*, the film stars Gary Cooper as a wanderer who comes to a remote island dominated by a Christian religious zealot. The character played by Cooper ends up championing the natives against the harsh and Puritanical discipline imposed by the religious fanatic on the island's traditional native mores.

In 1935, when socialites on the French Riviera and the United States found it fashionable to go to the beach in flowered brassieres and wraparound shorts that imitated the Tahitian *pareu*, in Tahiti women were forbidden to wear a *pareu*, as they had become considered indecent. Rather, they were expected to wear long cotton "missionary" dresses made in France.

Now history has come full circle and many Tahitians and French have reversed their fantasies and roles. When in the 18th century a dripping-wet and nude Tahitian beauty climbed aboard a French sailing vessel, all the fully clothed sailors were leering at the "naked savage." However, today, given the current European disenchantment with Christianity, it is more often the Pacific islanders who are the fully clothed and pious Christians and who can be found leering at the forms of the topless, sunbathing, neo-pagan French tourists.

Traditional Polynesians, after all, are practical. They know they can no longer live in the old way. For them, a person displays more *mana*, or power, when he or she acts more effectively, more practically. These days many Polynesians find it effective to act in the manner of their Christian conquerers. After all, if a young, unmarried Tahitian woman now becomes pregnant, her baby will not be welcomed warmly and raised by the whole village, as it would have been in centuries past. In addition, if today's Polynesian youth were encouraged to sleep around as much as their ancestors had been, they would probably all be infected with venereal diseases, which the Polynesians did not suffer from until contact with Europeans. Besides, today young Polynesians want to go off to a university and get a career, opportunities that did not exist in days of yore. If they became a mother or father at fourteen, as they had in the olden days, it would be difficult to go off to a university. Today many Polynesians find themselves divorced from most of their old, traditional ways, and with this sometimes comes a crisis of identity. Like Native Americans, many Polynesians feel neither really Polynesian, nor fully accepted as members of the cultures that conquered their lands. Finally, the fact remains that many native populations quickly dwindled upon the arrival of Europeans, due to disease. In light of all this, the Christianity that came to Polynesia along with the guns of the conquerors provided for many a refuge from the unnerving waves of "civilization" that have washed over them. Many of them now look back upon their former traditions as immature ways of being in the world, although there has been a Polynesian renaissance taking place since the 1970s. Ironically, the peace many Polynesians who have become

Christian feel in their hearts gives them a sanctuary from all the jarring and injudicious assaults to their lands and souls they have been forced to suffer at the hands of "civilization."

If you examine the sexuality of modernized peoples, you will find it much concerned with *images* of nudity—whether these images are from films, advertising, television, magazines or the Internet. Yet, as mentioned above, the minds of the early Polynesians were quite innocent of sexual images. They had neither pornographic magazines nor art—no Gauguin, and no hula girl postcards. Thus, whereas many minds in New York, London, Tokyo and Beijing are completely filled and fascinated with sexual images, early aboriginal Polynesian minds had no need for libidinal ideation at all. Their sexuality was not based on images. Their mental, psychological nudity allowed them a relaxed attitude toward physical nudity and sex. Whereas people in New York, London, Tokyo and Beijing become very concerned about body parts (men fantasizing about them, and women attempting to accentuate or augment them in various ways) the early Polynesians loved the whole person, body mind and spirit, not just a part of the person's body. Because the early Polynesians felt sex was entirely natural and because they had no *images* in their minds of mere parts of bodies, they had no fetishes and thus no perversions. That is a major reason why they were capable of developing a true and wise art of making love.

Furthermore, the love of the early Polynesians was entirely relational. After marriage, their sexual love was intimately connected with the entire life of their partner. They did not become overly fascinated just with a fraction of their lover's anatomy, but with the entire person and his or her life in the family and in the village. A mind filled with images and fetishes, however, is an isolated mind.

Such a mind is incapable of loving an entire person in relationship, because it invests all its erotic energy in devotion to a body part. The lovemaking of such a mind is always isolated and not really related to the actual life of the person it calls "lover." Such a mind can never enjoy a truly relational art of love, which takes a mind and heart free of images.

Even today the prevailing Polynesian image that dwells in the hearts of so-called "civilized" men—that of the bare-breasted and willingly amorous brown-skinned maiden—is not so easily washed away. This is because the image is a product of power. That power cannot be understood unless we look more closely at the first cultural interchange between Tahitians and Europeans.

When in 1767 the ship *Dolphin* approached the eastern coast of Tahiti, it was met by a Tahitian flotilla of 800 men in 100 canoes who had paddled out to greet it. The Polynesians were great navigators, however from time to time a Polynesian boat would be blown off its course and land on a strange island. The custom in Tahiti and in many other parts of Polynesia at that time had been that when a storm-tossed boat approached, it would be met with long speeches of introduction and then friendly greetings. The newcomers to the island were expected to give up all their possessions, including their boat, fishing gear, etc. in exchange for the hospitality, food and shelter they would receive. If they later wished to leave the island, their hosts would then provide them with a new canoe and provisions.

Thus, the crew of the *Dolphin* was greeted with friendly introductions and offerings of fruit and plantain leaves. The British sailors, in turn, offered knives, beads and ribbons in exchange for food. According to their custom, the Tahitians, considering the vessel theirs, then began taking nails, metal spikes, and other items they found on the ship. The sailors, however, not knowing the custom, interpreted the Tahitian's actions as theft and shot a cannonball over their heads. This gave the Tahitians the impression that their warm welcome had been ignored, and they would need to deal with the intruders militarily. However, they soon discovered that their stones and spears were no match for the *Dolphin*'s cannon, which could sink their canoes even at a great distance and lob shots up into the hills where the Tahitians had thought they had retreated to safety. Convinced that their fire-power was vastly inferior to that of the intruders, they feared for their future.

They decided to try another strategy. The chiefs ordered the canoes to be filled with attractive young Tahitian women, whose charms soon placated the sailors. In fact, this strategy of self-defense worked so well—creating a more genial form of cultural and economic exchange between the Tahitians and the foreign ship—that from then on, European ships sailing into Tahiti fired a cannon as a show of power. Is it any surprise they would be "warmly" welcomed? The Tahitian women's "welcoming" amorous embraces—which formed the basis of the Western image of South Seas women's sexuality—were bought at gunpoint.

Even today not that much has changed. The French, who took over Tahiti after a number of wars, instead of firing cannonballs over the quiet waters of Tahitian lagoons, display their power to the world by setting off nuclear explosions on Tahitian atolls, which they use as testing grounds for their atomic bombs. Possession of the Polynesian maiden's body and the power to represent her in images went hand-in-hand with the political conquest of the islands she inhabited. And the power of the bare-breasted Tahitian woman still beckons, for even though most of the inhabitants of most of the Polynesian islands have been "properly" dressed and repressed, thriving postcard and Gauguin print industries featuring bare-bosomed native women sprang up long ago, and endure to this day.

It seems Polynesians have learned to transform Western representations into cold cash. After all, tourism is a major industry in Oceania, where much entertainment is designed to cater to the centuries-old pinup mentality that others have of islanders. The nymphs of the pinups and postcards, however, are often Polynesian by citizenship only—not by blood. After all, many pure-bred Polynesians not killed off by war succumbed to European diseases, for which they had no immunity. The survivors tended to be hybrids, part Polynesian and part Chinese or European or American or Japanese.

The "*vahines*" beckoning on the postcards—whose photos perpetuate the myth of the *vahine*—are simply women with dark hair and a tan photographed on a Tahitian beach. They could be Thai or Chinese or Italian or Russian, and most viewers would neither know the difference—nor much care. The postcards and Gauguin paintings keep the myth of the bare-breasted hula girl alive, thus guaranteeing a constant influx of tourist dollars.

The astute reader will conclude that the image of the willing Polynesian beauty is a complete myth, in fact a myth created by the first European visitors to Tahiti, who simply held a gun to the hula girl's head. This image—so deeply fused with the reputation of the South Seas as bounteous with Isles of Love—actually has nothing to do with the aboriginal Polynesian art of love.

Art cannot thrive without idleness and an empty mind. Because good sex is an art, there can be no real sex, no lovemaking that explores the horizons of the sensual and the spiritual, without idleness. Postmodern, "civilized" men and women no longer know how to be idle. They are *producers* of things. Even the artists who live in cities are not really concerned with art. They—like the busy-bee workers from whom they pretend to be so different—are concerned with matters of little importance to art: production, promotion, gallery politics, museum hierarchies, and competitive rankings among metro-aesthetes. But all these insignificant factors constitute nothing more than the frame for art. They are not art itself, its dream, its body, its fragrance, and taste and passion. They are what remain after art is finished.

Similarly, "civilized" lovers are often concerned with a kind of production of love rather than with love itself. Seeking sexually to incarnate the images implanted in their minds from television, film, the Internet and print media, they become concerned with recreating those images and the production of orgasm. It seems to be the goal of much "lovemaking." Orgasm is like a gallery where lovers display the success of their union. Orgasm is the paycheck from the museum of having made love. Orgasm is an achievement, a frame that proclaims that lovemaking has been "artful." However, such "lovers" never stop to think what art of touching would blossom from a still mind, a peaceful, image-free, truly idle mind denuded of all thought, fantasy, fetishes and perversions.

"Civilized" people have forgotten that "success" in love, as in any art, is inversely proportional to hard work. For real art—whether sexual art, painting, sculpture—requires laziness, and laziness is fairly straightforward: It involves utter stupidity, abject dreaminess, absence of thought, staring at nothing, lolling about in bed for hours.

Is lazy loving even possible for civilized lovers?

Consider the experience of a typical Tokyo couple—Taka and Yumi. Before dawn, they are jarred from their dreams by the beeping or buzzing of their alarm clock. They drag their bodies into the bath-room, perform their morning ablutions, then make their way into the kitchen for miso soup, natto, rice and pickles. Hurriedly they rush off to catch the commuter train, wherein they position themselves like so many sardines in a can until the train arrives at their station, where they disembark, and walk to a building where they will endlessly toil like bees in a humming hive. Then, it is back to the train, home to bed, and the entire cycle begins again the next morning. On week-ends, they find themselves sleeping in—too exhausted to even think of erotic behavior.

Is it possible for them to practice Polynesian lovemaking?

Taka, with his charming wife, Yumi, checked into their room at a secluded hot spring in the mountains. Taka had been wanting to give Polynesian lovemaking a try for a long time. However, the couple's busy schedules had not allowed them time for any sex at all. Yet, he had read about Polynesian sex, and in his mind he imaged it as some-thing like a vacation—a peaceful place where he could escape the pressures and stress of his everyday life.

Their room at the hot spring hotel was not particularly spacious, but the bed was large and comfortable, and the room as well appointed. He lay down on the bed, placing his head on the pillow, and watched his wife begin to undress. He imagined with anticipa-tion their tranquil Polynesian embrace.

However, he awoke the next morning with his business suit still on. He was still lying atop the covers, but his wife slept beside him—in her Victoria's Secret negligee—under the covers.

He got up, took a shower, then went back to bed. His wife was beginning to stir in her sleep now. He curled around her from behind, feeling her soft skin and hair and the rhythm of her breathing. She was still sleeping, and after a short while, he too was dreaming peacefully.

When they awoke, he kissed her. "Let's try Polynesian sex!" he whispered, enthusiastically.

"If you want to do Polynesian sex, then take me to Tahiti!" she replied, jokingly. Then, she added, "We're in Japan now. Let's have Japanese sex!"

So, they went at it in their usual manner.

After it was over Taka lay there imagining what it would be like to have Polynesian sex, then he fell asleep, his body taking the rest it needed from the seemingly endless ringing of alarm clocks, rush of commuter trains, and hours of work.

In comparison to the busy Tokyo lives of Taka and Yumi, what happens on a Polynesian island is not much. In fact, it can be argued that Polynesia *is* laziness. The palms lining the beach greet the dawn in the same lazy manner they always have. Before dawn, if one looks far out over the black waters, a kind of pale place begins in the sky. Slowly, more paleness spreads. And the lagoon, which had been black, is after a while softened up to a rosy pink.

After another while, it could be said that the day begins. And the day is not very eventful. The entire beach seems to drowse in the sunshine and is empty and lifeless, or mostly so. At times a puff of trade breeze picks up, and the palm fronds sway. At times a coconut drops onto the sand. At times an outrigger canoe slips into the still waters of the lagoon and glides towards a passage in the reef. At times a woman languidly fills a basket with mangos. At times a brown and naked body slips into the lagoon for a leisurely dip, then emerges from the waters and is lost as it settles under the shade of a palm, to doze away the heat of noon.

All else is silence and slumber. Not a sound anywhere. Perfectly still, just as if the whole world were asleep. Only sometimes a set of waves breaks along the reef with a far, muffled explosion, and beyond the reef, the great Pacific, the majestic, magnificent Pacific, rolls its hemisphere-wide tide along, shining blue in the sun, silent and somnolent.

Days and months might swim by in such a silence, they slide by so quietly, smoothly and lovely. The very place induces a sense of rest and tranquility. The climate is of mid-summer warmth all year round. If a man and woman should embrace, they are in no hurry. Where bananas, coconuts and mangos grow everywhere and fish jump up into the outrigger canoe almost without coaching, it is easy to fill one's belly. Nor is love difficult to find. Seeing two men or women bathing in the lagoon, then stretching out in unconsciously voluptuous attitudes, chatting about yesterday's amours or their plans for tomorrow's was a common sight in Polynesia of yesteryear. In these isles lovemaking blossomed on a bed of silence, a stillness in which lovers had the leisure to explore subtle nuances of the art of touching.

When evening would fall, as it does so suddenly in these latitudes, in the patterns of light and shade woven by the moon, the shadowy figures of humans could be seen moving, the men singing and drumming as the women, naked to the waist, danced in rhythmical movements in imitation of the act of love.

In addition to the state of near nudity of the natives and to the tranquility of tropical islands providing an atmosphere for a relaxed approach to love—the cultural environment of the traditional Polynesians seemed, also, made for lovers. After all, the aboriginal Polynesians troubled themselves only about the needs of the day. They did not have to think about tomorrow. If it happened that a family found themselves short of food because of a bad crop, or unsuccessful fishing, or not being able to work because of illness, they did not have to worry. They had a kind of built-in insurance system that protected them in such times, because they could rely upon the support and generosity of neighbors whom they had helped in the past. Thus, the famous hospitality and gift-giving customs of the Polynesians formed a social network that protected everyone.

To hoard up riches for oneself was considered evil, but a person who gave away all that he owned was considered to be a paragon of virtue. After all, in a society that runs on solidarity and mutual help, the more generous a person is, the more generous people will be to him. Thus, there were no poor, unemployed or needy people in Polynesia of old. Nobody had to worry about housing, for their huts were produced easily and quickly from local materials. It was an environment where no one could possibly freeze or starve to death.

Because of the bounty of their natural surroundings, the Polynesians had plenty of leisure time and used it by dancing, singing, making music, playing games and amusing themselves in love. Poets and composers were continually creating new works, which gained popularity quickly.

Furthermore, the Polynesians perfected the realm of social interaction. So refined was their etiquette, so elegant their behavior, that it became akin to a high art. For instance, so intricate is the etiquette during the kava ceremony in Samoa, as anthropologist Bengt Danielsson pointed out, "that an orator must always take off his wreath of flowers before speaking, that the waiter may never turn the back of his hand towards a chief, that the handle of the wooden bowl should never be turned towards the girl who is filtering the kava," and so on. Thus, Polynesian life basked in both a natural and a social environment that was warm.

All these added up to create a way of life that is much different than that we find in modern cities. Whereas Asians and Europeans strive to accomplish something, to get things done, to attain a goal—the aboriginal Polynesians valued a comfortable, easy-going life with plenty of enjoyment. Whereas Asians and Europeans will try to do the best possible job and attempt to get the best possible result—the aboriginal Polynesians tried to get things done with the least amount of effort. Whereas "civilized" men will compete with each other ruthlessly, in Polynesia of old, life was based on cooperation and mutual help. In many "civilized" cultures the individual is important, in aboriginal Polynesia, the collectivity of the family or tribe was valued.

If in Chinese, Japanese and Euro-American societies people try to control their feelings, aboriginal Polynesians lived lives in which they gave immediate expression to all their feelings. If so-called "civilized" people value intelligence, skill, industry and reliability, the aboriginal Polynesians esteemed good birth, bodily beauty, hospitality and courage. Whereas so-called "civilized" peoples like to plan far ahead, the aboriginal Polynesians seldom gave a thought for the morrow.

And, whereas people in modern cities keep regular working hours, traditional Polynesians tended to let circumstances decide when it was necessary to work.

Such was the aboriginal Polynesian background for love: a lush tropical paradise overflowing with all the necessities of life, and should they somehow be lacking, a social environment that was based on the principle of mutual giving. Furthermore, the very personality was not rushed and anxious about time, but carefree and appreciative of the moment.

If the natural environment and social life were relaxed, so was everything about lovemaking, and the carefree attitude to love was taught even to visiting researchers, whom the natives would often consider to be sexually repressed. In fact, one naturalist who was visiting the Tonga Islands was curious about Polynesian mathematics. So, he asked a group of Tongan men to tell him the number system. His native informants told him all the numbers between one and one thousand, and he wrote them down. But then he persisted, wanting to know the numbers for a million, a billion, a trillion, etc. He did not stop to think that the Polynesian need for mathematical symbols was not as great as in Europe. The Tongan informants, having run out of numbers, however, were not dismayed. They admired his enthusiasm and—barely concealing their mirth—rattled off a whole series of sexual terms—words the man would never have written down in his own language—and did not stop until reaching 1,000,000,000,000,000.

Sexual attractiveness was very important in ancient Polynesia. Of course every culture has different standards for attractiveness. For instance, in much of the West today it is considered attractive if you are slim and tan, but for the ancient Tahitians it was important to be full bodied and as pale as possible. A sexually attractive person was thought to have more *mana* or power, so great lengths were taken to keep the body clean and make it attractive. Conversely, the more *mana* a person possessed, the more attractive they were considered.

Bathing was frequent. Polynesian women used herbs, massage and other means to enhance beauty. One of the most important herbs women used for their complexions was known in the Marquesan Islands as ʻeka (turmeric). Turmeric was considered sacred to a God know as Hai, and was used freely. It was believed that the odor of turmeric was sexually stimulating and that it had a beneficial effect on the skin. However, the Christian missionaries prohibited the use of turmeric, kava drinking, tattooing, dancing and sexual ceremonies—and today, turmeric is used only in cooking, as an insect repellent or a medicine for skin problems.

Many love cosmetics were used to increase sexual attractiveness and suppress body odor that might arise during the heat of love. Chief among these was coconut oil (*pani*) that had been scented with various flowers, but especially with the oil of sandalwood. Coconut and sandalwood are not only fragrant, but also cooling. Because the climate was always warm and lovemaking produces heat in the body, these oils helped lovers remain cool.

Flowers, as well, were worn for their fragrance, especially the *tia'e.* or *tiare* (*Gardenia tahitiensis*). This is the national flower of Tahiti (the one they give you at the airport when you arrive). It is also used for leis and floral head crowns, to honor people on special occasions such as birthdays or weddings, and at any kind of party. Many songs and dances praise the beauty and fragrance of this flower, and almost every traditional Tahitian medicine requires some buds of it. According to Jan Prince, writing in the *Tahiti Beach Press*, both men and women wear the flower, even today.

A man, *tane*, generally chooses a *tiare* Tahiti bud, while a woman, *vahine*, wears an open flower. They place the flowers behind their left or right ears, according to whether their hearts are taken.

When you wear your flower behind your right ear— it means you are *single, available and looking.*

When you wear your flower behind your left ear—it means you are *married, engaged or otherwise taken.*

When you wear flowers behind both ears—it means you are *married but are still available. Watch out!*

When you wear your flower backwards behind your ear—it means *follow me and you'll find out how available I am.*

When you wear a flower backwards behind each ear—it means *anything goes!*

When you see the young girl with flowers in her hair—it means *she's desperate, you'd better hurry up!*

Tahitian women, in days of old, used to pick fragrant shampoo ginger (*Zingiber zerumbet*), which grows beside the paths, squeeze it onto their long hair under a waterfall for a quick shampoo, redden their lips and cheeks using the lipstick plant and massage their body with *monoi* oil, prepared by soaking macerated *tia'e* (*tiare*) (Tahitian gardenia) flowers in coconut oil. Then they were ready for love.

Even today in Tahiti *monoi* oil remains a thriving industry. After all, *monoi* oil not only renders the skin and hair soft, but the fragrance of the Tahitian gardenia is relaxing and possess aphrodisiac qualities that make lovemaking heavenly.

Before the first European contact, Polynesians had no worries about venereal diseases. The aboriginal Polynesians were completely free of them. Nor did they have any worries about pregnancy. If a woman became pregnant, the entire village would help raise the child. Thus, many of the anxieties and worries surrounding sex in so-called "civilized" societies where simply lacking in aboriginal Polynesia.

Love, for aboriginal Polynesians, was a game. They did not have the concept of European romantic love, in which love for one's beloved is thought to be eternal. No traditional Polynesian lover would have dreamed of giving his or her heart once and forever. Rather, Polynesians tended to fall in love many times—and each time was at least as intense as the last. Nobody went around looking for the one right person to be with. In a society were everyone was almost the same, one looked for a partner who was physically attractive—pale, corpulent, and full of vitality—and skilled in the art of love and with whom one felt both physically and emotionally comfortable—those were about the only criteria if everyone was of the same religion, listened to the same music, and was of the same race.

Polynesian-style marriages were also supportive of a relaxed attitude toward sex, because in Polynesia nobody married simply for sexual reasons. Rather, aboriginal Polynesians married because it made life easier and more enjoyable. What few daily tasks that needed to be carried out—fishing, collecting roots and fruit, weaving mats, and other chores—could be doled out to different family members. Thus to have a family was to be able to lead a more relaxed life. Although the nobility liked to keep their blood line pure, and the parents almost always chose the marriage mate, among the lower classes there was much more freedom in choosing one's mate.

Nor was the institution of marriage in ancient Polynesia one that demanded absolute sexual fidelity. After the wedding ceremony and the couple began their married life, if the husband should have to travel because of war or a fishing expedition, both he and his wife were not expected to be sexually faithful during his absence. If the husband traveled to another island, his host there would offer one of his own wives to keep the man satisfied during his stay. Thus, in marriage, one could at times take the flower from behind the left ear and wear it behind the right. If the marriage began to wither, then divorce and remarriage were easy. After all, it was not difficult to find another partner with whom one would be harmonious. As already mentioned, in ancient Polynesia, everyone was of the same race, ate the same diet, listened to the same music, and shared the same religion and beliefs about family.

On the other hand, Polynesians did not simply leap from one marriage to another. Their marriages were often based on deep feelings. I paraphrase below from Robert Levy, who wrote of this in his thoughtful, sensitive anthropological inquiry into life in a Tahitian village, *Tahitians: Mind and Experience in the Society Islands*. In fact, I consider the young Tahitian man's thoughts to be a fundamental teaching on Polynesian lovemaking. This is because the basis of every relationship is the heart. The quality of the heart determines everything else: communication, lovemaking, and day-to-day living.

In Tahiti there were four major words for positive interpersonal feelings: *hina'aro, matau, here,* and *arofa* (the Tahitian equivalent of "aloha."). Young couples usually come together at first because of desire (*hina'aro*). As they remain together for a longer period, they become accustomed to each other (*matau*). They begin to feel love (*here*). Finally, they may decide not to separate because of *arofa* (compassion for the suffering of the other that separation would bring about).

In the 1960s, Levy asked a young Tahitian man if he and his *vahine* (woman) felt love (*here*) for each other. He said: "Yes, if we didn't love (*here*) each other, our life together in the house would not be going properly. For example, if only I *here-ed* (loved) Tetua (his *vahine*), and she did not *here* (love) me, then she would go and do the things that she desired, without taking me into account. And if it were the case, that it was Tetua who *here-ed* me, and I did not *here* (love)

Tetua, then I would not pay attention to her, I would only pay attention to the things that I wanted to. But the way it is, she *heres* (loves) and I *here* (love), and that's that. When things are like that, life goes properly for a couple. When you *here* (love), you have come to believe and trust with your body, with your thoughts and with everything, that this is your true *vahine*.

"And for example, in all kinds of activities that you think about doing, you request your *vahine* to do them with you. And, for example, there comes a time when you eat your meal in some place were you have been invited, and you arrive at that meal, and now you start to eat, and now your thoughts go to your *vahine* back in the house, because she is not eating that food that you're eating. And now, while you're eating, you have compassion (*arofa*) for her. You put aside a portion to take her in the house. That is *here* (love). That is the basic quality of *here*. You trust and believe in that *vahine* of yours. It is as if she were a parent for your household, for your way of living. That is what it means when Tahitians say *here* (love).

"Now there are some people who do not *here* (love) their *vahine*. He only desires (*hina'aro*) that *vahine* for someone to live with, but the whole ensemble of his thoughts has not come to be directed toward that *vahine*. That is the kind of person who goes into the amusement places. They enjoy themselves, pay attention only to their desire (*hina'aro*), and then they don't think any more about that *vahine* in the house. Those kind of people, it is said of them, 'They don't have *here* (love) for their *vahine*, but only desire…desire arising out of the body.'"

So you see that Tahitian couples came to love each other gradually. As teenagers they had a lot of freedom to explore. But as they became more mature, they settled down with one person and got accustomed to their partner, and felt love and compassion for him or her. In this way, they began to integrate physical, sensual love and emotional, spiritual love. I consider the young Tahitan man's thoughts to be a fundamental teaching of Polynesian relationships, because the basis of every relationship is the heart.

Another psychological factor that allowed Polynesians to be relaxed about love was the absence of what Freud called an Oedipal complex. According to this theory, a boy becomes sexually attracted to his mother and is hostile to his father. However, in Polynesia a child does not have just one mother and father, because children moved about freely from home to home. Polynesian children divided their affection between a large number of people in a village—all of whom were like mother and father. All those in the child's same kin-ship group were treated as one's near relations. In essence, there was no concept of a nuclear family. The very basis for development of the Oedipus complex was simply not present. When a child was born, he or she was handed somewhat carelessly from one adult to another. Often, the child would be nursed by women who were not even the biological mother. Thus children learned from infancy not to care for any one person too much. They did not expect a great deal from any given relationship. Instead of brooding internally and eternally on the qualities of one person, their concept of love was extroverted, realistic and carefree. Yet, the Polynesians were not libertines. Their good marriages were based on profound levels of feeling in the heart.

Still another factor contributing to a relaxed Polynesian attitude about love was the lack of contrast in gender identity. In the Tahitian language, for instance, one can listen to a person describing someone else for a long time, without learning whether the described person is a man or a woman. This is because in the Tahitian language, pronouns do not express the gender of the speaker or the person spoken about. Even the earliest visitors to Tahiti noticed the lack of gender contrast in Tahitian men and women. In 1890, Henry Adams wrote that Polynesian men and women are very much alike. And, as noted above, Gauguin, the famous French painter, noticed the same thing. "There is something virile in the women," he observed, "and something feminine in the men." Modern anthropologists have made the same observation. Moreover, the majority of traditional Tahitian names can belong either to a male or a female. Furthermore, there are many activities and chores that can be done either by men or women.

This lack of gender contrast in aboriginal Tahiti contributed to a relaxed attitude towards members of the opposite sex, so that they did not become some mysterious and distant object that can be invested with a lot of sexual tension, erotic fantasies and fetishes. Whereas Tahitians of yesterday blended and blurred distinctions of sexual identity so that seeing a person of the opposite sex was no big deal, in contrast, Euro-Americans tend to favor styles and displays of sexual contrast between men and women, for example, hiding, yet emphasizing various parts of the anatomy in order to create sexual-romantic tension.

The ultimate example of such a carefree Polynesian attitude about romance can be found in the behavior of the Arioi, a society of professional entertainers that sprang up in Raiatea in the 15th century in the Society Islands (now French Polynesia).

According to the Arioi, their society began when their god, Oro, decided to found a society of people who could devote their lives to singing, dancing and worship. In order to become a member of the Arioi, a man or woman needed to meet certain requirements. First, a member needed to be utterly attractive according to ancient Tahitian standards. Second, the member had to be intelligent, master of all the songs, dances and myths of the islands. Third the member had to be spiritual, showing evidence of being possessed by the god Oro.

Many thousands in number, the Arioi would travel from island to island. When approaching an island in their canoes, they were attired in yellow leaf skirts and red capes, their bodies glowing with fragrant oils.

Whenever the entertainers arrived on an island a great festival began that went on for days and weeks. All work stopped, and everyone became devoted to singing, dancing, making love and other amusements.

In the evenings, cool breezes heavy with the scent of tropical flowers would blow back their hair as the Arioi men and women swayed round-limbed, luscious-lipped, sweat breaking through the scented oils on their tawny skin. They circled and circled, voices rising in deafening waves, coiling and twisting, throwing back their heads wantonly, eyeballs reflecting a full moon rising over the dark volcanic wall of a valley, bodies bending upon swaying hips, arms rising and falling like waves with the animated rhythm of the dance.

The society of the Arioi helped maintain peace among the islands. It provided each island with professional entertainment and skilled sexual knowledge from the most intelligent and attractive people. It allowed artistically gifted and alluring men and women the chance to devote their lives to art, love and worship. Because the dramas it presented were satirical, it provided a form of social criticism.

How then can people living in modern societies aspire to the aboriginal art of Polynesian lovemaking? After all, it is neither possible nor desirable for everyone to start living a Polynesian lifestyle. Even the modern Polynesians find themselves hurried and stressed. But it is possible for you and your lover to learn how to relax and practice some basic principles of South Seas sexual communion. It is possible for you to discover a sexuality that avoids both the extreme hedonism of the traditional Polynesians and the extreme prudery of the missionaries who came to rule over those pure-blooded Polynesians who survived European contact. Finally, it is possible to make your mind and heart freer of images, so that you can integrate heartfelt sexual union with your spiritual life.

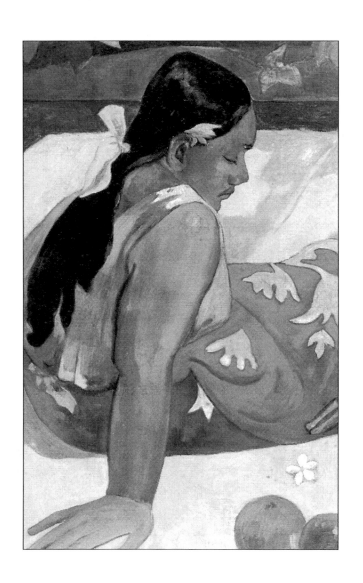

On Doing Nothing

*Paradise can be found, for without that possibility, why would
nature make the desire for it so intense and instinctive?*
– John Updike

*D*well in a plain and calm silence,
    With heart sensitive to subtle impulses.
Sip from the harmony of blended opposites.
And take wing with the solitary crane.

Like balmy breezes
trembling through your gown,
or rustling through slender bamboo,
a secret beauty will stay with you.

You come upon it by not trying deeply.
It fades away if you approach.
And even if it seems to take form,
It fades to nothing in a grasping hand.
– Ssu-k'ung T'u (837–908)

It may be that we have forgotten, fundamentally, how to look at the world. A boy riding beside his mother in the car beholds the countryside rolling by with the eyes of a child. He sees dark oaks illumined by the sun and green meadows splashed with mustard flowers and silent, golden butterflies. At the wheel, cell phone to her ear, chatting with her attorney or personal trainer, weaving between the trucks, the child's mother perceives the landscape only as an ambient blur.

Thus it may be that many of us are afflicted with a basic deprivation. Through constraints of time or the imposition of stress, we may find ourselves separated—as if by a glass wall—from Nature and even from the silent enchantment of simply being.

In our distraction, we may even have forgotten how fundamentally necessary and nourishing silence is to our soul. In our thoughts, we may even disparage the contemplative impulse as an utterly impractical calling. We cannot imagine ourselves wasting our time— if we had any—on meditation and contemplation.

Yet, silence bestows its rewards. It is silence that speaks to you when you gaze upon your loved one until your mental images begin to dissolve, your desires thin to nothing and you can no longer feel where you end and your loved one begins.

Inner silence bestows a blessed distance from the incessant demands of the world. Whether you are a CEO of a huge corporation, a mother or father, teacher or laborer—silence allows you to step back from the checkerboard of your daily responsibilities and contemplate the patterns of your life objectively, attentively and intelligently. In silence, you gain the ability to weigh the whole of a situation and to discover the importance of what before—in your haste—had seemed but insignificant detail. In silence, your heart ceases to strive towards things, your anxieties melt away, and the world—suddenly and mysteriously—unveils its enchanted ways before your wondering eyes. With a mind unclouded by mental images, you suddenly begin again to view even the simplest of things with the fresh vision of a child.

If many of us share a basic lack of silence—fortunately there remain sanctuaries where silence dwells—places devoted simply to being. There are places we may visit to restore our souls. As the travel brochures tell us, almost any tropical isle will do. Long before people set foot upon their shores, these islands flourished—serene, surrounded with placid lagoons, bathed in cool trade winds, and mute.

Islands abide in silence. And so abiding, they are revered, for they reveal the silence that abides within us. What voyager to an island has not felt the abysmal power of its stillness? Ultimately, words mean nothing on an island. Silently, islands refuse your names, descriptions and thoughts. Confronted with their uncompromising stillness you learn again to listen, to whisper, to touch and to feel.

The fine textures of silence on islands gently invite you to dive into the silence within yourself. Islands are like chapels that are open to people of every faith. And there are countless souls of every faith who have responded. Occasions have not been wanting for those who have crossed over the seas to set foot on their shores.

Islands do not speak to you with words of any particular creed. They speak to you with silence. That silence is you. It is you, yourself. Your very self. Your soul.

Yet, islands are only half about silence. After all, your soul no sooner—in silence—touches something immense, than it finds itself hurled back into time, refreshed and full of new vigor and visions for a hopeful future.

Silence, then, is for action. The silence of islands, after all, is creatively, alluringly alive, whispering sonorously to itself like the melody of a faint song. On peaceful mornings when dawn illumines the shapes of the palms and the fragrance of thousands of flowers is carried down the canyons by the offshore breezes, islanders begin to stir and stretch in the first rays of sun. As the sun climbs over the horizon, a man may be seen climbing a coconut palm, tiny wavelets may lap at the shore, birds may fight over a ripe mango. Yet, these sounds only deepen and enliven the silence, so that silence and activity begin to bow towards each other, to lose their boundaries and to blend together into one impulse of being.

In the late afternoons, when the light begins to soften again, filtering golden down through the palm branches, a vast calm settles over an island. Darkness slowly erodes the forms of trees and stones, and the landscape slides slowly, silently, irrevocably away—swallowed by night. Night fills the footpaths along the streams with nocturnal perfumes; below the canopy of palms, dappled moonlight quavers on the white sands; the stars peer down like a thousand thousand golden eyes; the stream—that far up the mountain cascades in a waterfall and flows into a deep pool—sings in the darkness, winding its way downward to a beach where waves kiss moon-illumined sands.

However, you probably do not live on a tropical island. You are probably not a brown-skinned island dweller, some languid Tahitian reclining on a pandanus mat, with calm eyes half closed, half-recumbent body almost limp, chin propped in hand, as relaxed as a cat dozing in the noonday sun.

In your busy and perhaps stressful life, you may feel you can never really enjoy Polynesian sex unless you can fly to some South Seas paradise and let your hair down for a while.

But all that is not really necessary. In fact, you do not really have to do anything. The good news is that—by doing nothing—you can become your own tropical island. The best thing overly busy people can do about their sex life is to forget about sex for a little while. After all, many couples, when making love, are used to doing so by pure muscle power. Otherwise they would simply collapse, because inside they are limp; they have no inner energy. They are exhausted. They actually need to simply give in to their fatigue and sleep. Their lovemaking is not supported by any inner vitality or keen desire.

Thus, lovers have first simply to be honest with themselves. That means they would have to allow themselves to admit their condition of fatigue or lukewarm interest. They would then realize that what they really need is rest—not sex. They are tired, and Nature is telling them to fall asleep. As long as they do not allow this, they cannot expect to change in any way. So when you feel like resting, learn to do it so fully and so skillfully that it is like curling up in the shade of a palm on your own tropical island.

And, in fact, you can become so relaxed, so at ease, so beyond the world that you feel as if you are in Tahiti, Bora Bora, Samoa, Nuka Hiva, hibiscus behind your ear, sipping cool coconut water.

How do you arrive on your inner tropical island paradise?

You will find it situated in the middle of an ocean—an entire ocean that moves within you—an ocean more vast than the Pacific, more subtle than any sea, an ocean you can dive into at any time.

Within a seashell's lips curls a song. It is the song of the sea of air. The shell is its shore. The same sea of air curls within the shore of your own body, and as it does so, quite naturally, its waves wash the shores of your soul.

You may have noticed there are almost as many teachers of breathing as there are of making love—many techniques, therapies, manipulations and systems. Some suggest concentrating on various energy centers within your body while holding your breath, others tell you when to inhale and how to exhale and in which rhythm. Such systems tend to make a god out of a technique, or of the breath itself. But if you are seeking a god or goddess it is only your true self, a silent, infinite being residing on the inner island waiting silently for you beyond the sea of breath.

The ancient Polynesians knew that the breath, like the ocean that surrounded them, was limitless and sacred. "Aloha" is a sacred word. One of its meanings is to allow more fully sacred breathing. In ancient Hawai'i, the traditional form of greeting was to touch foreheads and exchange breaths. "Aloha" also means love. How do we enter into the sea of our sacred, loving, breathing?

If breath is an ocean, you should not attempt to control breathing at all. For there are certain things you have no control over: High tide. Low tide. Waves surging in and washing out.

The waves of breath surge just as automatically as the waves of the sea. And the sea is not static. The great transformations of winds and clouds and rain and thunder and waves are always in a state of flux. Your waves of breathing are no different. Inhalation comes in to nourish the delicately porous shores of your lungs. Exhalation washes away all the used air. These are not controlled by any method. Your waves of breathing are utterly spontaneous, happening even when you sleep. And there is something mysterious about how this just happens. It has nothing to do with techniques, and the more you can set aside any techniques of breathing you may have learned—or any restrictions that may have happened to your natural breathing—the better off you will be.

Simply by sensing your natural breathing you can become your own tropical island. For the waves of your breath gently kiss an inner shore—an inner paradise that is utterly silent and tranquil.

To arrive there, follow no chart, no method. Simply float in your sea of breathing, sensing inhalation and exhalation, allowing the waves of breath to come and go spontaneously, as they will. For after all—when afloat on the sea you cannot impose a state of control over the waves, but can only allow them to come and go—up and down, up and down—as they please.

Thus, be not concerned with *how* to breathe, but only with *deeply* feeling natural breathing—becoming aware of this beautiful, oceanic guest who comes into you and revitalizes every cell in your body— and then goes. Simply sense these tides—with full feeling.

And I wonder whether it is possible—even while reading, that you can become so sensitive, so utterly permissive to breathing, that the air comes in and goes out just as it wishes—not as you have been instructed that it should.

Can you feel it? And can you feel how different it is just to be fully sensitive to your breath, without attempting to control or impose some technique?

Can you simply sense your breathing quite casually, not observing it from far away, not trying to influence it in any way, not saying to yourself that the rhythm of your breathing must be deep and rhythmical and regular?

Do you feel how the breath is changeable, how it will change to meet any situation? When you are swimming, running, walking, playing piano, lying in bed, kissing—or now—as you are reading, do you feel how your breathing will modify itself from moment to moment, mutating from instant to instant?

Do you sense how breathing is connected with your inner feelings? You might, for instance, notice that when you feel fear or insecurity, you hold your breath, but when you feel pleasure, you find your belly billowing out with deep, full breaths. So how can there be anything such as "proper breathing"?

As you breathe naturally—in and out—can you feel how your breath becomes more settled, and it becomes more calm, how your mind—usually busy thinking—becomes more calm as well? And can you feel how, as the mind becomes more settled, you sense more of your body, your feelings—your energy?

As you are sensing the ebb and flow of breath and the mind becomes more quiet—do you feel that the beauty of the present moment blossoms, and a wonderful shift from thinking to feeling begins to take place?

When you were a mere infant, your breathing was deep and spontaneous. As you inhaled, a wave of fullness, awareness and life surged down through your belly into your pelvic area and sexual region. If you watch a child sleeping you will see that with each breath the child's belly billows out, fully massaging and enlivening the area below the navel.

However, such an innocent state of breathing does not last long. As you grew, you may have been taught to feel embarrassed, tense or guilty about your genital area. You may have learned that the area below your belt is filled with things that are not usually talked about. You may have learned to pull in your belly and abdomen a little further, so they will stay out of sight. As a result, your innocent massage and stimulation of this area, through breathing, became disturbed. Instead of pulsing in rhythmic waves down through the stomach, into the pelvic region, giving it life, your breathing somehow had to find a new home, higher up, in your lungs. No longer does your diaphragm billow out fully when you breathe.

I wonder if now, while reading, you can allow your breathing to move sensuously, sweetly, in its own way, and discover what a delicately porous, tactile organism your entire body is as it allows breath to enter and leave. Can you allow it just to fill you and depart—without trying to lead it somewhere, without trying to manipulate it, but just allowing it follow its own nature? Can breathing be so free in you that when the air goes out, you do not try to help it along, but just let it go as lazily and quietly as it wants? And when it wants to enter you…can you permit it to come…and then to go of its own accord?

Can you allow breathing just to happen?

And as you go about your day—sitting, walking, working, looking at a flower, touching someone's hand, can you feel how breathing adjusts itself to whatever situation it meets? In this way, can you discover whether breathing is something static, or whether the waves of breath change every moment?

Can you make a quiet time, every morning and evening—when you light a stick of incense, and while it fills your room with its fragrance, sit comfortably with eyes closed—sensing your breathing for twenty or thirty minutes—simply letting the air flow in easily, as far as it likes, and then allowing it to flow out?

Can you feel that the incoming air feels cool in your nostrils, whereas the outgoing air feels warmer?

Can you merge with breath as it enters through your nose, the back of your throat, your lungs, your heart, your diaphragm?

As the breath goes in, can you feel yourself going in, also?

Do you feel how your rib cage expands and contracts as breath comes and goes?

Can you feel your shoulders rise and fall gently as breath enters and leaves?

Can you feel breath filling and swelling the area of your abdomen and your genitals?

As breath comes in, are you merged with it as it goes down, down and down into your abdomen?

Are you merely watching your breath as from a distance, or have you become one with it?

And do you notice that for a brief, subtle instant your incoming breath stops?

Can you feel how—for a fleeting moment—your breath does nothing at all? How there is no movement?

When breath is doing nothing, what is that moment like?

Can you sense this gap without trying to prolong it, but just noticing it?

And then, when the breath starts up again, can you become one with it, as it swells up through your lungs, throat and nose?

And as you merge with it, can you feel where it stops, outside your nose, and feel how, for a moment, the breath again does nothing—for a brief instant?

Can you feel how, for a moment, it is neither coming nor going? Can you feel your breath as it is completely still outside your body, in space?

So, when you are breathing, can you feel the breath not only as it comes and goes of its own accord, but also where the inhaled breath stops and does nothing, and the second stop, in the space outside the body?

Inhalation. Gap. Exhalation. Gap.

And I wonder if you can feel in those gaps, those stops, something subtle, something mysterious?

When breathing stops, does the mind stop also?

When breathing stops, do thoughts dissolve?

When breathing stops, does time evaporate?

As you sit, sensing your breathing and the gaps between inhalation and exhalation, do you notice that your breathing becomes increasingly more quiet, more calm?

Do you feel you are letting Nature do the breathing, and that you are just sensing the coming and going of the breath?

Do you feel how you do not have to do anything?

Do you feel how, sometimes, for a brief moment, when your breath is in the gap, doing nothing, all thought and desire and time will simply evaporate?

Do you sometimes—even for a moment—feel an extraordinary tranquility and peace dawning, as if you have become nothing—a very nice nothing?

In this state of nothing, you are mentally naked.

That feeling of a very nice nothing—that gap between the movements of breath—that absolute mental nudity, where there are no images in the mind—is your own private tropical island.

You will find that when breathing stops, even for a very brief instant—you do not stop.

You are still there. You are pure, radiant awareness.

Breathing has stopped, breathing is no longer there.

No inhalation. No exhalation.

But you are there, radiating the light of your own inner self.

This tranquil inner radiance is your own island that you can voyage to every morning and evening, before meals, when your stomach is empty.

And if a thought should come, do not worry about it, just let it be, and bring your attention easily, effortlessly back to your breathing.

If you journey to that island regularly, every morning and evening, you will find that as the weeks and months go by, the gap increases—your inner radiance and stillness increases. Your inner tranquility grows more and more calm. At first, it will be like just a small lagoon into which you might dip your toe to test the temperature of the water. But, as you experience that gap more and more, you will find that it will continue to grow so that it remains for many seconds, even minutes—naturally. The breath will come in or go out, and then the gap. And you will find that for a long while the breath stops, does not go out at all. All is silence and tranquility. Thinking has stopped. Time has stopped. There are no images in your mind. The entire world has evaporated. But you remain as radiant awareness.

In the gap, you will feel more and more relaxed, as if you are a brown-skinned Tahitian, sprawled out on a beach enjoying the sunshine, allowing your soul a chance to catch up with your body.

If both you and your lover can find your own inner island, and if you can voyage to that subtle island before you embrace, you will find that your loving will take on an entirely new quality. On that "inner island" your mind has no images, no fetishes, your love for your lover flows from the infinity of your heart to the infinity of your lover's heart. Because your love is free of images, if flows from whole body to whole body, and is not concerned with isolated body parts.

By entering your own private tropical island—in the gaps between the breathing—you both are entering the heart, you become love itself. Thus, you will discover a difference between merely making love and being love. The loving heart is aglow with the strongest electromagnetic field in the entire body. This field can be measured at a distance of ten feet from the body. As you enter the heart during meditation—and during Polynesian sex—this field of the heart becomes much more coherent, so that it begins to resonate with your lover's heart and brain waves. Then in an embrace with your lover you become one living sea of radiance.

Even if you are single and do not have a lover or spouse, the best way to attract a caring lover is to dive deep into your own heart. Not only will the magnetic field of your own heart become more powerful and coherent, but it will tend to attract a partner whose heart is also awakened.

You may say that you do not have time for twenty, thirty minutes, or an hour, morning and evening to sit and be aware of your breathing. And it is true that you may be simply too busy to take time for daily meditation. However, you *do* drive to work, you *do* take a commuter train, or walk or sit at a desk. Even during that time, in worldly activity, you can be aware of the coming and going of the breath, the subtle movement of the breath as it fills your lungs and abdomen. So if you are walking, you can feel the breath coming and going, and feel the gaps between inhalation and exhalation. You can do the same if you are riding in a commuter train, sitting at your desk, driving. And on the weekends, when you have time to sit, then you can sit and watch your breathing, especially before you embrace your lover.

If you do this—an entirely new world will unfold before your eyes. Perhaps for the first time you can look at your lover with "mental nudity," with a mind unclouded by images of any kind. In such a state the infinity in your heart can flow effortlessly and deliciously into the infinity within your lover's heart—though radiant whole-body loving union.

And remember: "You come upon it by not trying deeply."

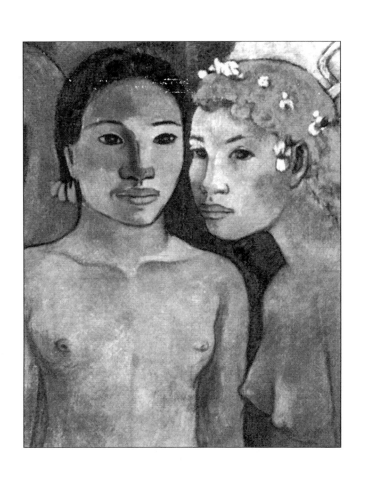

On Touching

I am the poet of the Body;
And I am the poet of the Soul.
–Walt Whitman

The evening has arrived.
   Beside the bed glows the golden aura of the candle.
Within your heart you feel an even fuller glow.
It fills you sweetly, overflows your limbs.
Your lover snuffs out the flame—
runs his fingers through your hair.
Your body is enfolded in infinite night.
His touch comes to you as in a dream.
In darkness,
he looks at you
with the eyes of his hands—
with the moist eye of his mouth—
with the glowing eye of his heart.
Within your body hidden waters awaken.
Your breath
—a veiled wind—
quickens.

Your breasts
—two little doves with fluttering hearts—
are cupped in his hands.
Your breasts—
two little moons –
rise and swell—
illumining your night.
Your breasts are silken in their softness.
His fingers swim through the waves of your body.
Your body enters the river of his hands.
Your breasts swim in his hands like twin fruits
—ripening.
He takes your breasts
into the hollow of his mouth
—he takes your breasts
into his very heart.
He tastes in your breasts
the song of your own beating heart.
He touches you with flower touch—
you moan with star pollen.
He touches you with feather touch—
you moan with soft mango.
He touches you with fire touch—
you moan with warm honey.
He touches you with rainbow touch –
you moan with rain song.
He touches you with stone touch –
you answer with hidden lightning.
His touches—

lighter than air—
lighter than kisses—
open the petals of your body –
They uncover there
another nudity
within your nudity –
They discover
within your body,
a secret body
of honey water –
They carry you inside yourself
to your island of silence.
Your soul opens—
a white moon blossom,
fragrant—
tremulous.
(*after Octavio Paz*)

Or—does your body respond, but your heart and soul remain untouched, isolated, closed?

When your senses join together with those of your lover, do you really touch emotionally and spiritually what you touch with your body?

Or do you and your lover—in the force of your passion—merely attempt to touch what you cannot really embrace?

Do you—like a monk and a nun who have taken vows of

chastity—actually abstain from deeply touching each other—spiritu-ally, emotionally—at the very core and heart of your being?

If you cannot truly touch one another's heart, does not this inabil-ity at the very heart of your desire, of your need and of your loving truly constitute your appetite?

Do you devour each other—while never really tasting what truly nourishes your souls?

∼

Conventional sex—based primarily on stimulation—assumes that touch cannot arise from within. Rather, conventional lovers assume that their sense of touch must be stimulated from without, physically, by stimulation of sexual trigger points.

In conventional sex, stimulation—in all its forms—seems both necessary and sufficient for touch to reach fulfillment.

Yet, when your touching is based solely on stimulation of sexual trigger points, when the energy can be aroused only through a touch from outside, upon a surface of your body—then it is desire that is stimulated—not love. And the energy of desire accumulates within your lower body as sexual tension. You tense increasingly around this tension, focusing on it.

This energy grows in force like a river. But it does not find a way to circulate within your whole body—from the area of the genitals up into the emotional center of your heart and into the spiritual centers in your head. It remains localized in the clitoris and the head of the penis.

Because your energy does not circulate, it gradually becomes more and more concentrated, tensing your body until the energy is expelled. At first you express this accumulation of delight and energy through moaning, sighing and breathing heavily. At a more intense level, your voice will cry out, scream or sing. At an even higher level of intensity your energy will throw your body into movement—and then—when your body can no longer accommodate the accumulation of energy that has built up—your body will expel it, through tensing muscles and waves of orgasm.

However, is touching about the end of the embrace—about orgasm—or is touching about the embrace itself? Is your orgasm the fulfillment of your touching? Or does the fulfillment of your touching depend instead on how much delight you and your love are capable of discovering and circulating within your united bodies—for hours?

Can you and your lover navigate your hidden currents slowly, endlessly exploring, swimming through the ancient waters of your body: your loins of water, your lips of water, your eyes of water, your waist of water, your rivers of heartbeats, your dark river of hair, the luminous rivers of your heart and spirit?

Or does your capacity for experiencing delight soon arrive at a crisis, a spasm? Do you tense around your erotically focused energy? And does your energy take on form, accumulating in your lower body and becoming expelled down and out, through orgasm—depleting vitality and extinguishing the force of desire?

Do your genital organs have only a reproductive function—which requires orgasm—or do they also have a social and energetic function—as conduits of energy and ecstasy?

Do you, in assuming that touch can come only from outside, overlook the hidden possibility of inner touch, of deep feeling?

For love is not made in the same way that one makes a painting or a bed or a meal. Love is not something that can be worked on, polished, created by an act of will.

Loving is total surrender—a sacrifice of your entire self—body, mind and heart.

If love were something that can be made, that is an art—then it is not the lover—but something the lover has produced through an act of will.

Suppose you go to an island where the natives have never seen electrical gadgets. You show your radio to a tribesman. You tell him it is for making music. So, he begins to bang it on the ground. Maybe he beats out a pretty complex and exciting rhythm. But he is misconstruing the nature of the instrument. Your body is like that radio. If you treat it simply as a percussion instrument, then you will enjoy merely a conventional level of sexual experience. The radio plays its own music, from within itself, because it is in contact with an ocean of energy that is invisible, subtle, not obvious, and all pervading.

If you are sensitively in touch with the energy field of your lover, you will feel that love is not something you make, in a percussive manner, from outside—but something like the merging of two inner oceans—and that you and your lover must be quiet—at rest within yourselves—in order to really sense and bathe in the merging currents and surrender to the luminous tides.

What if the real fulfillment of your touching is not in orgasm, but within the heart? What if the limit of your touching is not external—throwing off energy—but internal—circulating and sharing energy?

In the previous chapter you explored a space between your breaths where you can enter into the heart and discover the silence that shines there.

What you found there is a limitless secret that dwells within a sea of silence with no external boundaries, an absolute innerness that is untouchable by thought and images. Yet, at the very heart of your heart—on your island of inner silence—you will find an offering, a sacrifice—because your limitless heart will overflow, abandoning itself to the heart of your lover. Your heart goes beyond itself— reaches out and touches the heart of your beloved. When this happens, infinity touches infinity. You know that you really do touch spiritually what you touch physically.

This is why it is important that you explore the subtle inner realm of touch—in the place of silence within your heart— through meditation, before exploring the outer realm of touch through sexual contact.

By learning how to rest within yourself—within the heart—your "tropical island"—you can explore the inner realm of your touching, where your heart flows beyond itself to include and embrace your lover. Only then can you truly know yourself and touch your lover deeply, circulating your energy endlessly.

Thus, sensitive lovers make love in a way that involves not only the genitals, the lower body and the senses, but also the heart—the element that is able to blossom from within itself and reach beyond itself to touch the heart of one's lover.

You may have noticed, in an emotionally vulnerable moment, when you and your lover drop the masks of your personas and show each other your true, deep feeling—maybe with many tears—that at such a moment sex becomes somewhat unimportant—because you and your lover feel no distance between your hearts. When you both feel truly in the heart—the necessity of orgasm can, for a time, lose its force.

In your truly heartfelt embrace, what takes place is not really restraint—but a spontaneous balancing of your external touching and stimulation with your inner fullness of the heart. This point of balance dwells at the pivot between stimulation and stillness—between the stirring of your passion and your sense of repose.

Otherwise—if you remain too much stirred by external stimuli—you will become incapable of an awareness of your heart. You will remain merely at the mercy of external touch. This will disturb the natural stillness of your heart.

Stimulation actually divides. If you notice when you stimulate your lover, you will find that your lover becomes less and less aware of you and more focused on his or her own desire.

But if you and your lover are resting within the heart—such resting does not divide, but unifies. Both you and your lover can fuse with one another in luminous relaxation, peace and freedom.

When stimulation overwhelms—you and your lover expel your energy and may not really touch each other's hearts.

When resting in your heart overwhelms—you and your lover dissolve into one another and may forget about sex.

Thus, sensitive, playful lovers swing back and forth between these two extremes: playing at the pivot between stimulation and stillness. This integrates the sensual and the spiritual.

The beauty of Polynesian sex is that it fully embraces both sensuality and silence——holding them in balance. The selfish drive to orgasm, with its focus on the self, threatens to pull you apart from your lover—setting you in opposition to one another, and depleting your inner energy. That force is countered by relaxing into your heart, which makes you and your love feel as though you are one unified body and spirit—strengthening your inner energy. When you learn to blend these two forces, you reach the fulfillment of your touching.

Thus, learn to abide on your inner island. Then, explore with your love the magic realms between stillness and stimulation—be at play within the seas of calmness and sensuality—sensitive to both receptivity and activity, to what is solid and what is empty, to what is form and what is formless, using sensitivity to nourish the inner feeling and energy.

When such sensitivity blossoms, it can open for hours. Light will gather around you and your love. You will grow in brightness—drifting between purity and passion—at rest in the current of love, bathing together in the flooding stream, immersed in its waters.

In this chapter I list some guidelines for Polynesian lovemaking. Because we have found it is almost impossible for busy couples in the 21st century to have enough inner tranquility to enjoy Polynesian sex, I have added one thing to the suggestions for exploring Polynesian-style loving: Before making love, close your eyes and voyage to your inner "tropical island," which exists in the gap between the breaths. Otherwise, you may find yourself just using these teachings to prolong conventional sexual contact rather than integrating your deepest silence with your deepest touching.

It is important that you view these suggestions as suggestions, as invitations for exploration of new possibilities, rather than as rules. After all, the mind tends to rebel against rules. There is a huge difference between: "I AM FORCED to do something" and "I DISCOVERED something really great." If your attention dwells too much on rules and steps, then you may find yourself focused on HOW to do something rather than on the flow of WHAT you are doing. Therefore, I have written this entire book not as a series of rules, but as suggestions for explorations, for discovering something new, for finding out about yourself. Explore them playfully, seeing where they lead you, and never force them on your lover or yourself.

These suggestions for Polynesian lovemaking follow:

1. Have intercourse not more often than once every five days. On other nights, sleep together, body-to-body, an art in itself, without contact between the sex organs.

2. On the fifth day, preparation for making love should include at least twenty or thirty minutes of meditation, of closing the eyes and voyaging to the gap between the breaths, your "tropical island."

3. On the fifth night, foreplay takes at least an hour. Caress, embrace, kiss and bite each other, until you both are electrified.

4. With actual penetration, lie united and motionless for at least half an hour, or even longer, before starting any movements.

5. If you experience orgasm, continue to lie together for a long time. This will allow you to equalize and blend into one ocean the streams of energy that have been awakened in your two bodies.

Below, I have listed these steps again, with commentaries and detailed explanations.

To really make love unhurriedly, with awareness and sensitivity, takes time. But you should not be aware of time when you are in an embrace.

Thus, Polynesian sex is not something that you can do as a "quickie," before rushing off to work, or for fifteen or twenty minutes before you go to sleep. If you are rushed, if you are in a hurry, you have allowed the element of time to creep into your lovemaking—and this element of time will not allow love to fully blossom. If a sense of time enters your lovemaking, if you do not allow yourself the leisure to feel the full unfolding of pleasure—you may feel you *must* have an orgasm just in order to convince yourself you have achieved something.

True lovemaking, however, requires that you forget about time, and this can be done only if you have set aside at least a couple of hours to fully relax into love, allowing it to fully blossom.

1. *Have intercourse not more often than once every five days.*
   On other nights, sleep together, body-to-body, an art in
   itself, without contact between the sex organs.

This guideline insures that you have some inner energy, vitality, aliveness and desire built up, so that your lovemaking will not be just two fatigued bodies going through the motions of stimulation. How closely you care to follow this guideline will depend on several factors: the intensity of your desire, your age, your degree of health and whether or not you are experiencing orgasm when you make love.

During these five days, do meditation every day. Get enough rest so that you really feel inner energy within yourself. Massage your lover when you can, becoming aware of his or her energy. Do Tai C'hi or yoga. These will help you to dissolve tension and stress that block your energy and will give you an awareness of energy flows within your body.

If you give your body a rest for a few days, then your inner energy and desire will build up so that you can enjoy lovemaking that is not just physical, but a real exchange of *energy and delight*.

Sensitivity should be the guide. You can learn to be sensitive to your own inner energy, so that you will know when you are really making love with inner energy and desire—and when you are just going through the motions. It is good if you and your love are able to communicate about this and reach an agreement on frequency—or even better—become so sensitive to each other that you will sense when mutual desire is strong.

Many of the teachings on Polynesian lovemaking esteem motionless, skin-to-skin contact. Early in the twentieth century anthropologists learned about societies where every infant was carried against the mother's bare skin for much of the day. In such societies, the infants, who were constantly being touched, were much more relaxed than children who did not receive much skin-to-skin, maternal contact. Further studies showed that the bodies and minds of infants deprived of skin-to-skin contact did not develop naturally.

Such full-body contact lessens bodily and sexual tensions. The prolonged and motionless full-body contact between lovers during Polynesian-style lovemaking, and on the other nights when they are not actively lovemaking, creates a sense of tranquility and relaxation. When the lovers do begin making love actively, they do so from a relaxed, calm state of being. Their calm body-to-body togetherness naturally becomes less concerned with erotic stimulation than with delighting in already present sensations of soulful union. On the nights (and days) they do not make love actively, they are still, resting in love, being in love.

This is in sharp contrast to much of the lovemaking in so-called civilized societies, where prolonged skin-to-skin contact is more rare and where sex often begins from a tense body and mind that require quick orgasm to relieve the stress.

2. *On the fifth day, preparation for making love should include at least twenty or thirty minutes of meditation, of closing the eyes and voyaging to the gap between the breaths.*

You will be sexually what you are emotionally and spiritually. The quality and depth of your union is simply a printout of the quality of your inner life, your heart. Therefore, as I have indicated in the previous chapter, the best thing you can do for your sexual life and your relationship in general is to forget about sex for a little while. Learn how to dive into your heart during meditation, and then make a habit of doing it every day—and especially just before making love. If you can do that, you will spontaneously find that when you are making love all the waves of stimulation, desire and passion are energized and surrendered into the sea of your own blissful consciousness.

If you and your lover have learned how to enter the vastness that resides in the gaps between the breaths—then you will both be able to radiate that vastness to each other during your embrace. You will find your loving embrace becomes a spontaneous sacrifice of body, mind, and ego, and that the entire sexual function will relax into the current of inner vitality and awareness. Then, your energy is circulated and felt in the whole body, which itself surrenders to an infinity of bliss.

It is excellent if you meditate, do Tai C'hi, or do yoga with your lover on a daily basis. In this way the field of energy between you will grow stronger. But if your lover has no interest in meditation, then giving your lover a full-body massage before having sex will help your lover relax and help the energy to circulate between you.

3. *On the fifth night, foreplay takes at least an hour. Caress, embrace, kiss and bite each other, until you both are electrified.*

If you have meditated before you start kissing and caressing, every touch and nibble will flow out of inner silence. Your sense of touch will be more subtle. Each caress will blossom on a bed of effortless, relaxed and expanded awareness. Simply bringing this expanded awareness into your love play will transform it.

After meditation, just feeling the presence of your lover can be enough to make the mind and heart enter back into a meditative state. Sensual contact with your lover can itself be quite meditative, because the mind focuses easily on pleasure. After meditation you are able to listen to and be inwardly attentive to the finest stirrings and tender impulses of your energy and feeling as these blossom from stillness. You will find yourself opening to deeper levels of sensitivity, sensuality and communion as you continue to make love in a relaxed manner. You will become attentive to each touch, each pause, each movement, each breath.

It is helpful if both you and your lover can be aware of breath, just as in meditation, because it is your breath that distributes your stimulated energy throughout your body so that you do not tense around it. So, when your lover is caressing you, do you feel your breath is involved in the area that is being caressed—absorbing the stimulated energy and distributing it to the rest of your body?

If you have meditated first, then your caresses will tend to begin quite gently and lovingly, infused with much silence and feeling. And at this time—if you are a man—it is especially important to apply this post-meditative lovingness to your lover's breasts—perhaps beginning with just cupping them very gently, or breathing on them. This is because her breasts are so intimately connected with her heart that she naturally has a deep desire to have her breasts touched and loved tenderly. The more lovingly they are touched, the more she will open, ready to absorb your love.

Most men do not understand how much breast stimulation can arouse a woman, and that the longer such stimulation lasts, the better. Men should keep in mind that the sensitivity of breasts will change from year to year, from day to day, from moment to moment. At times they may become too sensitive to even approach, except with the subtlest of touches. Therefore, always begin gently—neither touching nor sucking nor nibbling too aggressively, as this may be too much for your love, and even cause her to withdraw her body from lovemaking—just as your penis would want to draw away from over-aggressive touches.

Given the sensitivity of breasts, and the different touching preferences of each woman, if you are a woman you can help your lover by conveying to him how you prefer to be touched on your breasts and nipples. If this communication takes place, then you will not have to silently endure a type of stimulation you do not really welcome.

Men should keep in mind that after their lover becomes more aroused, her breasts may hunger for stronger touch.

If you are making love to a woman, the more you touch her breasts with great love and tenderness—the more your own heart will become awakened—as well—simultaneously. However, keep in mind that some women feel no sensitivity in their breasts at all. When real affection and communication exists between two lovers, they naturally relate to each other their preferences.

In general, the way to awaken the woman's vagina is not—at first—through the genitals directly. Rather, in the depths of the night, if her heart is awakened thorough loving attention to her breasts, hands, wrists, eyelids, little hairs at the back of her neck, the darkness between her breasts—her genitals will slowly begin to blossom as well.

Simply by bestowing such attention on his love, the male will become sufficiently aroused for love in the Polynesian mode. Therefore his lover should be sensitive to his level of excitement so that she does not put him over the top before penetration.

4. *With actual penetration, lie united and motionless for at least half an hour, or even longer, before starting any movements.*

In the conventional approach to love, after some time of what is called "foreplay," the man usually enters the woman and begins thrusting. The thrusting will grow in intensity and become faster and faster.

However, in the South Seas sensuality, after a prolonged period of caressing, when you and your lover's bodies have become electrified with passion, and then penetration takes place, remain motionless—or nearly so—for about half and hour, moving only enough to maintain the male's erection.

After the swimming of two bodies—two waves—within the sea of night—the male searches out his lover, reaching where she has been waiting for him in her rose-wet cave. He enters, but the two bodies come to rest. The arms and legs rest, closed around each other. The lips rest. Lingering moans soften and fall like petals in the softness of night.

Two bodies entwined—in union—flooded with still luminosities.

In the Polynesian approach, your bodies, which are now flooded with the magical biochemistry of love, join fully together genitally, but then come to rest. In this silence, the aroused energies, which have congregated in the area of your genitals, are then diffused throughout your whole body, mind and heart. When this happens, you feel a deep sense of union. Your two beings—through deep rest—become joined together at profoundly deep energetic levels.

Many men have expressed surprise that by doing such a simple thing as resting within their lover—after arousal and penetration—their lover experiences tender feelings of fulfillment. Often, they say that they had been under the false impression that they must do a lot in order to satisfy their woman, only to find that by doing almost nothing, they accomplish almost everything.

An etheric resonance begins to vibrate between you and your honey as you come to restful surrender in each other's arms, holding each other gently. Your bodies will feel oceanic, almost formless—and in your hearts you will feel a sense of fullness and wholeness—calm, and harmonious. You will be brimming with a tranquil physical pleasure and emotional satisfaction that is luminously limitless.

This is because as you do less and less through your will—your spirit does more and more. The spiritual dimensions of sexuality really begin to unfold when you begin to relax in your intimate embrace. The more you relax, the more you become aware and the more you feel. Relaxing down into your sexual energy allows you to diffuse and absorb it—inward and upward in a glorious current of energy and light—rather than experiencing it as it builds up into a peak and is released downward and outward.

Then—after such a period of motionlessness—when you and your lover's bodies begin to move again—instead of moving more and more rapidly—move more and more slowly, only enough for the male to maintain an erection.

After some time you may feel the need for orgasm, and you may feel yourself tensing around that feeling and focusing on it. At this point you have the choice either of indulging in genital orgasm or of transcending genital orgasm altogether, through whole-body diffusion of the sexual energies.

Even if you agree with your love to enjoy genital orgasm, you can still benefit from the technique of being sensitive to the pivot between stimulation and stillness—between passion and repose. For by doing so you will not only discover a way of making love that will last for hours, but you will also feel that making love will enhance your vitality. You may begin to feel you can begin to contemplate an intensely pleasurable current of energy moving through the entire nervous system and body—a current not thrown off through orgasm. You may feel your vitality actually increasing rather than being discharged, and you may find this vitality nourishing the entire nervous system and system of endocrine glands.

If, on the other hand, you want to explore Polynesian lovemaking without orgasm, keep in mind that it is not about cutting off the animal part of yourself in the area of the genitals. It is not about saying, "Oh, I'm spiritual now, so I'm not going to have orgasm during sex." It is about feeling those energies awaken in your lower body and surrendering to them as they circulate throughout your whole body.

Usually, if you indulge in conventional sex, you exploit your sexual ability to have an orgasm, as a release mechanism. After all, every day you may encounter resistances to your desires. You may become tired and stressed. You know that if you can stimulate yourself to the point of orgasm, you can forget all that—at least for a moment. Therefore, you may tend to think about sex often. Some researchers have found that both men and women think about sex at least once every few minutes.

But is all this thinking about sex an entirely practical preoccupation? After all, a person who is sexually active experiences orgasm for only about twenty seconds each week. That is about ninety seconds each month, or eighteen minutes each year. However, conventional orgasms, in these brief spaces of time, rather than circulating the life force, eliminate it, as if it were a waste product. Therefore, unless you are very young, when this type of orgasm is indulged in frequently, over time, it will prove to have a devitalizing effect.

Yet you may find yourself exploiting sexuality in general, and orgasm in particular, in order to escape from your tensions, stresses, and frustrations. It may be for you the only occasion in your life when you feel intensely connected with your inner sense of energy and aliveness, as if everything else is just killing time.

Thus, you may seek to gain a partner who, with the minimal amount of effort, you can manipulate into providing you with sex, ending in orgasm. And yet—such sex may not really fulfill you. It may not bring you lasting peace and contentment. It may be an intense pleasure for a moment, but then it fades. It depends upon stimulation, genital tension and a spasm of genital release, not whole-body feeling and love. It is a solution that you may use to escape, even for a brief moment, from pain, fear, tension, sorrow, and anxiety. It is touching that does not really touch.

However, with Polynesian lovemaking, it becomes possible,

instead of throwing off your accumulated genital energy through conventional orgasm—to circulate it throughout the entire body so that it nourishes the glands, the emotions and the spirit.

One of the natural processes you can use to accomplish this is simply moving more and more slowly, rather than more and more rapidly. Or you can simply stop and remain still for a while. Another natural process you can use is breathing. You have seen how you can become aware of the gaps between your inhalation and exhalation to find a limitless ocean of silence within your heart, to create a Polynesian sense of tranquility before you make love. And when you are in a sexual embrace with your lover, you can still remain aware of the breath—and the gaps between inhalation and exhalation.

Even in a sexual embrace with your lover, can you breathe naturally, just letting your breath come in and go out as it wants—not trying to control it in any way?

Can you ask yourself: What is my breathing doing?

Are my breaths long, even, relaxed and calm, or is my breathing disturbed?

Am I trying to control my breathing, or do I allow each inhalation and exhalation during sexual play to occur naturally, completely free of any strategic control or emphasis?

Is my sensitivity to each inhalation and exhalation, my feeling of relaxation into the process of breathing, as profound and alluring as my sensitivity to my genital contact and sensations?

And as I inhale, can I feel my belly expand?

What does my belly feel like?

Is it hard, soft, relaxed?

Can I feel my belly moving with my breath?

What is happening there?

Can I feel it living as my breath enters and leaves it?

Does my belly seek its own shape?

And is my belly involved with breathing?

Can I feel breath entering my belly sensitively?

Does my breath find its own way in my belly?

Do I feel my breath penetrating sexual regions?

Do I feel the breath when it encounters the built-up sexual energy that has amassed in the lower body, below the belly?

And what happens when I move the pelvis forward and backward, slowly, as I make love?

Do I feel my breath as it merges with and dissolves the accumulated sexual tensions, diffusing them to the rest of my body?

How does my breath feel in the region below my navel?

Can I feel the breath entering the region of my sexual organs?

What does it feel like when my breath enlivens that area?

Do I feel the energy wants to go down and out my sexual organs?

Do I feel a glow or warmth in my sexual organs?

I wonder if I can feel the breath move behind the sexual organs, into the region at the base of my spine?

What does it feel like there?

Can I feel what my breath does there?

Maybe I feel the base of my spine glowing?

Now, can I feel the breath, again, in the area of my sexual organs? Where does my energy want to go?

Down and out?

Now if I invite the energy to move around to the base of the spine again, do I feel it wants to travel up the spine again?

And if so, do I feel that energy moves into the region of the heart?

Now just let breathing find its own way.

Where does it want to go?

What region does it want to penetrate?

Where does it want to move?

Do I find it bringing sweetness wherever it goes?

If you become aware of your breath and your energy—in this way—as you are making love, moving your awareness back and forth between your accumulated genital tension and your breathing, your spine and your heart—you can become aware of the pivot between stimulation and stillness, between passion and repose.

After enjoying Polynesian lovemaking for some time—you will feel your body becoming "rewired" so that automatically your life energy circulates without being thrown off through orgasm. You will begin to feel your sexual energy spontaneously drawn up the spine towards the heart.

However, if you are just beginning to practice Pacific passion, then you may find you need to resort to means that are more physical in order to stay within the pivot zone. The following techniques are helpful in this regard.

As you feel energy accumulating in the region of your genitals, energy that would ordinarily lead to orgasm, you can relax the entire body, ceasing or slowing down its motions, and breathing into the sexual energy until it dissolves and is diffused into whole-body awareness in the region of the heart. You can simply rest within the arms of your lover until a sense of relaxation and peace and heartfelt union returns. You may feel a sense of etheric, magnetic resonance between the deep energies of your bodies. After resting in this way, you may or may not feel like resuming movement and stimulation again.

This is a good time to change positions, because by playfully engaging in different positions during lovemaking, different parts of the body, especially of the penis and vagina, are stimulated. Changing positions thus helps to redistribute and circulate accumulated sexual energy to different parts of your body—prolonging pre-orgasmic play. Because different parts of the penis and vagina correspond to various organs—when the penis and vagina are stimulated from different angles by changing positions—glowing health is the result. Thus a varied choreography of sexual embraces not only ensures prolonged pleasure, but augments health, a glowing complexion and happiness.

Some different positions from the Marquesas Islands, where French painter Paul Gauguin resided, are as follows:

TITOI KAUKAU (INTERCOURSE ON THE SIDE)

Both you and your lover lie on your sides, facing each other. The position was also known as *haka ka'aka* or *haka na'ana* (in Hiva Oa dialect), which means 'in the gecko-lizard manner.' Taoist sexual manuals assert that this position has therapeutic values. If the woman lies on her right side, keeping her lower leg straight, but bends her top leg backward, while he faces her and penetrates her—the internal organs—especially the liver and kidneys are strengthened. If on the other hand, the woman lies on her left side, with her left leg bent as far toward the back as possible, while keeping her right leg straight, it will heal broken bones, bone marrow diseases, arthritis and leukemia. The same position, but with the woman on her right side and her right leg bent back was used for blood vessel problems, including varicose veins and hardening of the arteries. High or low blood pressure related to blood vessels was also said to be helped by using this position.

PATU HOPE (STICK THE BEHIND)

The woman kneels down or bends over the horizontal-growing trunk of a palm tree, receiving the male in her vagina, from behind. This position was also known as *titoi ihorave* (Horse Intercourse) or *titoi peto* (Doggie Style). But the Taoists called it "Tiger Style."

HAKA NOHO (SITTING STYLE)

The woman sits astride the man's lap, facing him. She does the moving, but he helps her by moving her hips and buttocks. Taoists called this "Crane Style."

HAKA PE'E

The male reclines face upwards, the female sits astride him, on her knees. The Taoists used the position for many problems relating to the blood, including those of blood pressure. It was said to be good for anemia, low blood pressure, poor blood quality and blood clots.

TAMURE

Circling movements during lovemaking—from the

Tahitian dance of the same name. Upon arrival in Tahiti, almost anyone would become instantly fascinated with the way Tahitian women move. They look like they feel inside as if the very fact of their physical existence is a great joy to them. Dancing to polyrhythmic Polynesian drums has a lot to do with it. Even when not dancing, the women move seductively—but once the drums start pulsating, their knees bent low, their thighs rhythmically exposed, their shoulders back, and their hips rolling fast and smooth, the women move like sensuous goddesses. They have the ability to move their hips in rapid or slow circling motions.

One can easily imagine them straddling their lovers, red hibiscus in hair, their black flowered *pareu* loosened over their thighs, their hips tracing lazy, almost imperceptible circling motions, as their hands move in the gesture that means "clouds gathering over mountain."

Make love as many do in traditional cultures, where lovers do so for hours by making similarly languorous hip motions, enjoying each other in mutually relaxed positions. Instead of rushing headlong for a quick peak of stimulation in the "missionary position," which is suited for pumping and bumping and reproduction, be sensitive to your inner energy and enjoy gentle, never-ending waves of life coursing through your body.

A second method you can employ is to apply pressure with the fingers, just behind the genitals, near the perineum. Both the male and the female may do this. This is a nerve center, and pressing there will considerably lessen the urge toward orgasm.

A third method, from traditional Polynesia, was called *'ami'ami* in Tahiti, and in Hawai'i, *'amo'amo*—the "wink-wink" of the vulva. The technique was used in sexual intercourse and creates a perfect balance between sexual stimulation and stillness, and was also known in India's Tantra circles and by ancient China's Taoists, who called it the Deer Method.

Taoist sages noticed long ago that deer enjoy strong sexual abilities. Observing deer, they saw that the animals exercise their anal muscles when they wiggle the tail. After seeing this, the Taoists begin doing something similar. They found that the Deer Exercise develops all the tissues of the sexual organs. Second, they discovered that the exercise draws the energy upward through all the glandular and energy centers in the body, transmuting sexual energy into spiritual energy. Third, they found the exercise increases the flow of blood and energy in the abdominal region. This flow of blood and energy helps to transport the energy of the sexual center to the rest of the body. The fourth benefit is that the Deer Exercise enables lovers to prolong sexual intercourse, because it moves up and distributes sexual energy. Further, the exercise exercises the prostate gland and female sexual organs, so that they remain healthy. Over time, the exercise builds up mental power and inner tranquility, as well.

If you are a man you may do the *'ami'ami* while standing, sitting or lying down. All one needs to do is tighten the muscles surrounding the anus and draw them up and inward. When done properly, it will feel almost as if air is being drawn up the rectum as the entire anal area is drawn inward and upward. Tighten and hold as long as you can comfortably. Then, stop and relax. Then repeat the anal contractions. Repeat this as many times each day as you can, without feeling discomfort. Over time, as you practice, you will find that you are able to hold the anal muscles tight for longer periods. It can prevent and correct many sexual problems, including premature ejaculation, wet dreams, impotence, and so on.

If you relax your anus when you thrust into the vagina and squeeze the anus as you pull out, your endurance will be greatly improved. Done during intercourse, it moves the sexual energy upward along the spine.

If you are a woman you may do *'ami'ami* by tightening the muscles of the vagina and anus, as if trying to close both openings. Try to draw up the rectum, inside your body, further contracting the anal muscles. When done properly, this will feel as if air is being drawn up into the rectum and vagina. Hold these muscles tight for as long as you can comfortably. Relax and repeat as many times as comfortable. If done regularly and correctly, you will notice increased sensitivity and an inner glow that spreads from your lower spine into your heart and head.

A fourth technique of prolonging pre-orgasmic pleasure in traditional Polynesia was known in the Marquesas as *nini'e* (scratching) and *ki'i naku* (pinching) and *moma kai* (biting). The scars and bruises from such love play were proudly displayed and were also a way of marking one's territory. If one of the lovers was going away on a journey, they would both mark each other as much as possible. Scratching, pinching and biting also served to sharply draw the attention and energy away from a focus in the genitals. So, these actions could not only heighten passion, but also prolong it.

As you explore Polynesian love over time, you will notice you need to take less and less recourse to these physical means and that orgasm is transcended instead simply through full-body awareness.

Polynesian sexual play is based on your having an intimate relationship. Your sexual play will then transcend orgasm, conserve life energy and vitality, improve health, promote longevity and augment mental and spiritual clarity and tranquility. You will begin to feel profoundly peaceful both during and after lovemaking.

Perhaps you will have already been practicing some form of yoga, meditation, Tai C'hi, hula, or belly dancing. If so, you will be intimately familiar with and sensitive to subtle levels of body sensations and energy flows during your yoga, meditation, Tai C'hi, hula or belly dancing. Not only do such practices produce energy flows in your body, but these energy flows are not felt only in your genitals, but felt all over your whole body and can be quite subtle. Often your awareness can become so effortlessly focused, so absorbed in these sensations that it dissolves your physical, material sense of your body. You actually dissolve the materiality of your body and pass beyond it. When you feel the sense of having a physical body simply vanishes, you may find yourself floating in waves of energy and light. Eventually, even those waves and luminosities may fade away and you may enter into a great vacuity impossible to describe. If you are a yogi, meditator, Tai C'hi practitioner, dancer or lover and pass beyond form and physical sensation—you have entered into the perfection of your art—no matter what it may look like from the outside.

The two first words of a famous Chinese poem by Wang Wei describe this experience of transcending the physical dimension. The words are *kong shan*. They mean "empty mountain." In the same way that it may seem impossible for something as massive as a mountain to be "empty," it may seem difficult to go beyond the physical body—but yogis, dancers and lovers have this ability.

When you have learned to transcend the physical body and enter into an intimate embrace, you may discover that when your sexual energy builds up in your lower body, it suddenly and quite forcefully rushes up the spine in a powerful wave. As this wave of energy courses upwards, it may shake and vibrate your body quite uncontrollably. When this happens, your movements in love can become extremely passionate, but they are not done willfully. You have simply surrendered to the powerful flow of energy that is ascending the spine—and this energy accomplishes all that needs to be accomplished. This wave of energy will bring about a kind of spiritual-emotional orgasm that shakes your entire body, but is not accompanied by ejaculation in the man.

After experiencing it, you will naturally wish to remain resting within your lover's arms, because a sense of whole-body fullness and diffusion of delightful energy will have replaced the sense of concentration in the genitals. In such an embrace, the motive of orgasm relaxes and the motive of sexual intercourse itself comes to rest in ecstasy. The impulse of desire relaxes and you can rest in mutual bliss and love.

If you have some experience of energy ascending the spine—then such an embrace can sometimes be brought on willfully. The man, atop the woman, uses his arms to push his upper body up, in a kind of effortless cobra pose. Then, only the genitals of the two lovers are in contact. As the genitals are then the only point of contact between the two lovers, they become the conduit of the tremendous energies accumulated within them. The lovers may feel that their genitals become especially sensitive and electrified. Because the body of the man is in the cobra posture, which facilitates energy rising up the spine, the accumulated energy may start spontaneously rushing up the spine in waves, throwing his body uncontrollably into passionate movement. Because he is united with his lover on a deep level, her energies will join in the same current. Her body, also, will begin surfing effortlessly in its waves. What they have experienced is an orgasm of the entire body, mind and spirit. The man will not ejaculate—and when the waves subside, they will find immense sweetness in simply resting in each other's arms.

After continuing in the practice of Polynesian lovemaking for many months, tensions within your body, especially within your genitals, and petty, reactive emotions and mental images will tend to evaporate from your life.

However, because Polynesian lovemaking involves the physical body, to adapt to it fully takes time. It is a gradual process. It is not really a technique. Simply, your sensitivity as a lover awakens—over time—as you make love with increasing awareness. It is an ongoing and spontaneous process of refinement. You cannot expect to be operating in one way sexually for all your life—focusing on fantasy and orgasm—and then change suddenly overnight. So, it is best if you adapt to it slowly rather than suddenly adopting it.

The first thing you may want to do is to meditate daily, and live within a loving relationship with growing emotional intimacy. This means you and your honey must sacrifice all your private and reactive emotions—by talking about them with each other. Further, it is best you mutually agree to pursue Polynesian lovemaking and be mutually cooperative when you are doing so, helping each other to learn and explore its possibilities together. After all, you are launching into a complete re-education of your nervous system. And this re-education takes place not through thinking, but by making love with awareness. This awareness will show you that making love is not about the goal of the embrace—but about the embrace itself.

In addition, sometimes fantasies that are mutually acceptable should be permitted in your sexual play. The very fact that your hidden fantasies are being shared with your lover and that all this varied love play is taking place in relationship to one another undermines the very foundations of self-possessed, self-absorbed, relationless pleasure. Over time, your sexual play will become more and more about intimacy and relational love. As intimacy grows, your capacity for enjoying Polynesian lovemaking will increase.

At first, do not try to suppress orgasm while making love. In fact, if you do, you may feel that an excess of sexual energy will build up. It is not really circulating to the rest of your body and it needs release. In such an instance, simply continue with conventional sex until orgasm.

When adapting to Polynesian lovemaking without orgasm, do so with awareness of breath, an awareness of the accumulation of sexual energy in the lower body, and an awareness of love in the heart. Pivot back and forth between genital stimulation and heartfelt rest. Instead of having an attitude of doing sex, have an awareness of being in sex and in love. But at first, use Polynesian lovemaking only to prolong the period of lovemaking prior to orgasm. Then fully enjoy orgasm.

After you have done this for a few weeks or months, next explore what it feels like when you stop having orgasm. Finally, after more time, you may feel the entire motivation for orgasm decreasing, and that your vital energy will spontaneously ascend your spine and circulate.

As you become more sensitive to your energy and more mature in the art of Polynesian lovemaking, you may find that when you make love, genital tensions simply do not arise. Further, you may find that general body tension and even body movements are not so necessary to feel full pleasure. You may also feel that your body at times feels formless, without boundaries, insubstantial. You may find that during love, your breathing is greatly relaxed, spontaneously. At times you may find that your breath may even stop as you transcend thought and enter a spiritual state with your love. You may find that your mind is empty, with no images during lovemaking, and that your body and heart feel full of boundless bliss.

5. *If you experience orgasm, continue to lie together for a long time. This will allow you to equalize and blend into one ocean the streams of energy that have been awakened in your two bodies.*

It is important not to separate quickly from your lover. While making love, you have been weaving a beautiful, subtle fabric of energy. If you break away from each other too quickly, it tears that fabric.

The benefits of languorous love are many. Whereas conventional sex is generally brief, and culminates in orgasm, lazy love can be prolonged for hours and does not necessarily involve orgasm. In conventional love, pleasure is felt mostly in the region of the sexual organs. During slow love, the entire body and emotions are enlivened. The energy that flows downward and outward during the orgasm of conventional sex, creating a degenerative exhaustion of vital energy, instead flows upward into the whole body, all the glandular centers and the heart, rejuvenating them. After conventional love, you may feel like separating, because the flame of desire has been extinguished by orgasm. However, after slow love you and your lover remain vital, sexually interested and sexually interesting, fully capable of intense sexual activity. There is no sense of depression following lazy love—only a sense of radiance and relaxation.

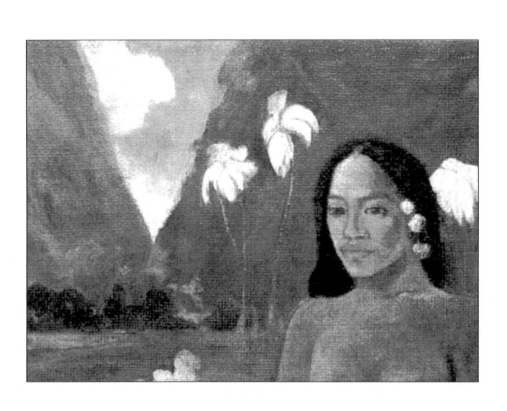

The Secret Valley

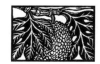

*I*f you were to approach Tahiti by sea, as did the early Polynesian navigators in their catamarans, the first thing to greet your eye—far across a vast expanse of rolling blue—and after the solitude and isolation of a long sea voyage—would be a smear of light visible slightly above the horizon. Depending upon the hour, this rising luminosity could take on the pink pallor of dawn, the golden glow of evening, or the whiteness of noon, as it illumines the crown of clouds hovering about the highest—but still hidden—Tahitian peaks.

A few hours later, these dark and jagged summits, themselves, would begin to rise into view—and then gradually the massive slopes of volcanic mountains would slowly unveil themselves. It is not until you are almost upon the island, skirting the reefs and their exploding surf, that you would see high valleys laden with flowers and golden fruit, and—after slipping through a pass in the reef—feel the calm of the silent, opalescent lagoons and begin to make out on shore the brown bodies of the Tahitians moving in their long, sensuous gaits, or relaxing gracefully in repose upon a porch. You would then smell the fragrance of breezes laden with copra and unknown floral scents from deep, hidden valleys.

Those light-infused clouds crowning the peaks, which had at first appeared only as a glow just above the horizon, will now be floating serenely, veiling fractured peaks, which now tower high above you, the muffled roar of the breakers, and—if it is evening—wild bodies dancing in abandon to the throb of music. You realize that Tahiti is a mountain that has risen from the bottom of the sea. A good part of the land is almost vertical—and the serene, light-infused clouds are a part of throbbing Tahiti—yet always apart from it.

These clouds gather up the moisture from the shores and valleys, wafting it upwards to their cool heights and then sprinkling it down in cool showers that refresh the hot and busy lives so far below.

Your own body, in love, is similar to a Tahitian isle. Like the clouds that adorn the volcanic peaks, you are capable of delighting in a serene and cool detachment that rains down showers of energy upon your loving—even while your sexual organs are joined in playful union with those of your partner.

The secret to enjoying spiritual bliss even when you are deeply engaged in a loving, sensuous, embrace lies in your ability to be sensitive to subtle energy flows within your body and the body of your lover. In the chapter "On Touching" you have seen how you can circulate energy from your lower to higher energy centers, through being aware of the pivot point between heartfelt stillness and sensuous stimulation. Whenever your energy begins to amass in the area of the genitals, through stimulation, you can simply rest and relax into the heart—radiating your feeling of love into the infinity of love within your partner's heart.

Such a method is natural if you and your honey are deeply in love and have some awareness of your heart energy. Not everyone, however, is in such a relationship. Perhaps your sexual partner is someone for whom you may not feel deep love at the moment—or you may simply be the type of person who is more independent and distant—

even in your sexual relations. Perhaps you have difficulty with really feeling heartfelt energy. Perhaps you feel neither especially caring towards your partner, nor do you especially wish to feel cared for. Perhaps you harbor a deep fear of becoming emotionally dependent upon your partner and an actual terror of being hurt—as you may have been at another time in your life. You may feel unlovable, unworthy of being cared for, and may actually select mates who are neither nurturing nor view you as worthy of being treated equally and lovingly.

If you are such a person, a method of slow loving that relies upon a degree of surrender to the heart energy might simply prove boring. However, you are fully capable of enjoying great depths of Polynesian lovemaking—through another method.

If you are capable of feeling your body as a Tahitian isle—where the waters of the valleys, instead of flowing down into the ocean, instead circulate up the slopes to the serene, cloud-illumined summits, and then cool and condense to rain down and refresh the activities in the lower altitudes—you will have entered into a great secret.

In fact, on the Southwestern point of the island of Tahiti Nui you can find the magical grotto of Mara'a. Here a stream flows from the mountainous interior of the island, filling a cavern with waters that are cold, clear, fresh and midnight blue. At the mouth of the cavern maidenhair ferns, blue morning glories, mosses, and a rainbow of other blossoms, wet with dew, beckon. Even through the current flows outward to the sea, it seems as if something draws one into the grotto, an allure almost impossible to resist. Within, the dark cavern opens to a vast dome, where thousands and thousands of water droplets drip down into a pool of deepest blue. According to Tahitian tradition, this pool is the door to Paradise.

The teachings state that if you dive into the pool at Mara'a and swim against the current beneath the blue waters toward the mountains, you will enter a secret, blessed valley abundant with all the fruits of Polynesia. In this valley, the teachings say, no one grows old or becomes ill. And whosoever enters that valley will find dwelling there—the gods.

Your body is like the island of Tahiti at Mara'a. Just as the waters of the grotto flow outward to the sea, similarly, your sexual energy and fluids have a tendency to surge downward and outward. So, the method relies upon reversing this outward flow of your sexual energy. Instead of streaming down and out, it circulates from the area of your genitals, backwards towards the perineum (a spot between the genitals and the anus), and then it curls up around your sacrum to the area of your kidneys. This area behind your genitals is your secret valley. Once your energy enters there, it will have a tendency to ascend up the length of your spine to the space where your skull meets your spine, and then into your head, as if the waters in the secret valley are carried up the slopes of the interior mountains. Then your energy curls down again along the front of your body, over your heart and abdomen, down through your genitals, and down again through the secret valley of your perineum.

The blessing is to be aware of your circular flow of energy—rather than upon sexual thoughts and images. A good way to practice this is through meditation. With inhalation, feel your breath moving from the sexual organs and your perineum, around your sacrum, up your spine into your kidneys, then up the full length of your spine, into your head. Your tongue curls gently back, so that it just touches the roof of your mouth. Thus, when exhalation takes place, feel your energy moving down from your head into your tongue and then down the front of your body, through your heart and stomach, into your genitals. Then comes inhalation, and your energy is drawn up again.

Another way to practice this is to imagine the circle of energy moving down the front of your body and through your genitals and perineum with inhalation, and then up through your tailbone and spine to your head with exhalation.

The most important point is the flow of energy from your genitals to the perineum and around your tailbone to your sacrum. This space is like the secret Tahitian valley at Mara'a. To enter here is to enter a paradise of spiritual-sexual pleasure and health. As your energy is moving through this secret valley, it will help to perform the 'ami 'ami (wink wink) contractions, also known as the "deer exercise," as described in the previous chapter. This will help your energy to be pumped up the spine rather than flowing down and out through your genitals.

Once your energy moves through the secret valley, you will feel it building within the region of your kidneys, and as you continue to breathe, it will be drawn up into your head. When it reaches your head, you may have the experience of your body disappearing and your awareness being absorbed in a sea of light and bliss that has no boundaries.

Then, with exhalation, you will feel that light and bliss raining down the front of the body towards the genitals, where the cycle of energy begins anew.

Once you have practiced this during meditation, you can then practice it during self-stimulation or while making love with a partner. Once the circle of energy becomes complete and natural, you will be able to make love for hours with your partner—falling more and more deeply into increasingly radiant pools of welling energy. Any time you feel yourselves approaching orgasm, merely stop moving, but continue feeling the circulation of energy in this circle.

Once you and your partner have learned to feel this circle of energy within your bodies, it is time to learn how to include each other in the circulation. This is done is a similar way to circulating energy within your own body. However, instead of moving the downward-flowing energy through your own tongue, you feel it move into the tongue of your partner. So, for instance, if you are the man, you feel the energy moving from your head into the tongue of your partner as you kiss. You then feel it moving down the front of her body, into her vagina, and from her vagina into your penis. Then you feel it flowing through your genitals, through the "secret valley" in the area of the your perineum and past your anus, up your spine, and into your head again.

If you are the woman, feel your energy moving from your head into your partner's tongue, down the front of his body, into his penis, and then into and through your vagina, where it flows through the secret valley of your perineum, around to your sacrum and up your spine into your head again.

If you and your partner dally in this loving embrace you will begin to feel energies playing between you in many different patterns as you find yourselves enveloped in a sweet nimbus of energy. As you persist in this form of intimacy, you may find that your vital energies begin to spill into your emotional centers and open your hearts. When this happens, you will be capable of engaging in the mode of Polynesian lovemaking considered in the chapter "On Touching."

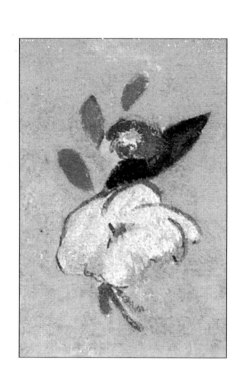

The Silence of The Hummingbird

*T*he stony trot of a couple of burros, the clang of church bells, the sounds of car motors and radios—all were drowned in the thunder of the locomotive as it hissed, wailed and screeched down the slopes from Mexico City. Santiago—dressed impeccably in a white linen suit—took in the passing countryside: white towers of churches in town squares, colors of fleeing parrots, stands of trees seething with crows, a barefoot girl standing quietly among tall sunflowers.

The spring break was just beginning, and Santiago was looking forward to visit with his University of Mexico classmate Enrique, who lived in a small village in the mountains above Vera Cruz. Santiago had been raised in a large colonial town, could claim some European ancestry, and felt it would be amusing to see how rural Mexicans, rich in Indian blood, lived.

There was no glass in the train windows, so that with each passing kilometer the rushing air grew warmer and more humid, and Santiago was soon sweating profusely. He had nothing to wipe his brow with but the back of his hand, and it was not long before his discomfort forced him to take off his suit jacket and unbutton the top of his shirt. Two seats in front of him a peasant was taking a sip from a canteen, and Santiago was beginning to regret his choice of clothing.

It seemed to Santiago as if the train would never arrive, because as it chugged slowly to a stop at each little town, he began to think that each little town looked exactly the same and he began to grow impatient—not only with the progress of the train but with the very idea of Mexico. After all, Santiago surveyed his environment with two stunning blue eyes. His grandfather had been Spanish, and these facts had always led Santiago to regard himself as being a cut or two above your run-of-the-mill Mexican. And so, bored of looking out at the Mexican landscape as it rolled past, Santiago began to daydream about that proud man—his grandfather—and of how he wrote beautiful poetry and created beautiful designs on fabrics at the textile mill where had worked, and of how he drank and laughed with his artist friends until late in the evenings in smoky cafes, and of how he had married the town beauty—Natalia. But especially Santiago daydreamed of how his grandfather had spoken with Natalia, in their entire marriage, only five times.

It was this fact that captivated Santiago whenever he thought of his grandfather—and just as the rumblings and clangings of the train drowned out the sounds of the church bells and rivers it passed, the thought of his grandfather's silence drowned out the sounds of the train. Santiago found himself thinking of his grandmother—her frail but still beautiful white face framed with black lace—explaining that his grandfather had spoken each of the four times after her labor when she came to him with the newborn child in her arms. She would hold up the child toward him, and he would say only "What color are the eyes?"

When Santiago's grandfather was a young man he first noticed Natalia in school. He had later taken her as his wife. It was at her fifteenth birthday party that she had first danced with him. And for her, that had been it. His movements were as fluid as a river's, and in his arms, she felt herself floating.

After marriage, his life with her had been one of silence. He loved her. She loved him. But he directed her only with his eyes. He spoke to her only with his eyes. He seduced her, scolded her and succored her only with glances. And in that silence they had learned to drink from deep wells of being.

After they had lived together for a few years, one day Natalia hired an old widow to help with the housework. When Santiago's grandfather had come home from partying with his artist friends he saw the old woman. Then he went to his wife. He told her he did not like old women, and that she would have to let her go. This was the fifth and last time he had spoken to her.

And so Santiago had long thought of his grandfather as a god-like being, and he wished that he, too, could marry a beautiful woman, live with her in silence, and seduce and scold her with only his eyes.

When the conductor barked out "Acatlan," Santiago was soaked from head to toe.

The first thing Santiago noticed about the pack of young men at the depot—dressed in white *playera* shirts and pants—was that each wore a leather belt, a holster and a pistol. Enrique greeted Santiago with a sweaty handshake, and Santiago, tossing his head and laughing, pointed to his friend's pistol and joked, a little nervously, "Expecting *banditos*?"

The men smiled at Enrique, and Enrique looked at the men and smiled. Then they all laughed. Enrique's fingers moved to the butt of his pistol. He withdrew it slowly from its holster, held it up, examining the sheen of the barrel in the strong sunlight. "Nope, amigo" he grinned. "We just use these to shoot at monkeys that get into the orchards."

"Oh!" laughed Santiago, still a little nervous, slapping Enrique on the back, "Monkeys!" The other men laughed, too, and Enrique picked up one of Santiago's bags. He looked at Santiago standing there in his wet shirt, holding a suit jacket in his hands.

"Expecting *el Presidente*?"

Everyone laughed again, and then there was a moment of awkward silence.

"Hot?" asked Enrique.

"Yes, yes…I'm soaked. Is there somewhere I can take a shower?"

"Come," Enrique said.

Santiago picked up his other bag, and the group walked together down the dirt street of the village. The buildings were of many colors: bright yellow, pink, red—and many were two or three stories high. On the second story there were large balconies with ornate iron railings. Almost everyone greeted Enrique and the men as they passed, and the girls looked at the young dandy who walked with a white suit jacket slung over his shoulder, and who moved like a puma.

Beyond the last building Santiago saw that the dirt road entered a mango orchard. Even in the shade, it was still hot as they walked along in the dappled light. On the other side of the orchard, the road led to a line of greenery and a bridge. Beyond these, the horizon was a broken skyline of mountains.

The men walked down the road to the bridge. When they reached it, their boots sounded on the wood planks. They stopped and leaned out over the railing. The water flowing down from the mountains was clear and looked cool. One of the men cleared his throat and spat into the water. Santiago heard voices coming from beneath the bridge. He leaned out and looked under. A path left the road and circled around under the bridge. There in the deep shade next to the water, it looked cool, and there loitered men and boys—some swimming, some just sitting nude in the shade, some smoking cigarettes. Beyond the reedy shallows the current was swift, and he could make out the dark forms of large fish—finning silently.

On the opposite bank, beyond the reeds, and muted by distance— the shrieks of girls could be heard above the sound of the river. From a distance Santiago could see them moving among the reeds, and a few girls swimming in the open river.

"This looks great!" said Santiago.

"OK, let's jump in!" Enrique said. He picked up one of Santiago's bags. Santiago picked up the other, and the men began walking down the path that led under the bridge.

The window of the guest room looked out over the mango orchards, towards the river. On the wall was a niche with a small statue of the Virgin. Santiago was resting on the bed, chatting with Enrique, when a dark-haired beauty of about twenty years of age walked into the room.

Santiago and Enrique stood up. "Santiago, meet Rosa, my sister."

Santiago looked into her luminous brown eyes. He nodded warmly, but did not speak.

What surprised Santiago was the moment he saw her, it was as if he had seen green thunder. Enrique's mother brought in a candle, placing it in the niche in the wall, and Rosa stretched herself out on the bed where he and Santiago were lounging and began to talk with Enrique as Santiago listened, talking on and on about a place on the coast, far away, where the palm trees grow and the blue sea crashes on the shore and the white sand stretches on for miles and miles. They talked of the dark shadows of fish in the river and of the arrow snakes in the jungle and monkeys in the mango orchards and of a blind old man who plays his guitar sweetly in the town square, and their own shadows danced in a garden of muted flame as Santiago found himself drowning in the humid swellings of syllables rising and falling between Rosa's laughter and the naked flashings of her eyes.

Sometime later the three of them fell asleep, surrounded by night and the immense breathing of the forest.

In his dreams it is always a mysterious woman Santiago dreams of. In his dreams he always takes her to the coast. They follow a dirt road to a small fishing village. Santiago arranges with a fisherwoman in the town to bring them some breakfast the next morning. Then he and the woman take off their shoes and walk in the sand, far down the beach, where they are all alone.

Night comes with its thousand thousand stars and the waves crash on the sand.

In the morning, the Mexican woman brings a basket containing sweet tamales, beans, fish, salsa and mango. She smiles a little when she sees the patterns the two bodies have made in the sand during the night. Then she leaves.

The mysterious woman takes a palm leaf from a tree, kneeling in silence before it, she spreads it out. Silently, as if upon an altar, she places the tamales, the beans, the fish, the salsa and then the mango.

Santiago sees himself kneeling on the other side of the palm leaf. They take their meal in silence.

The next day Santiago was floating in the current, beyond the reed beds, around a turn in the river, when out of the blue of a whirlpool Rosa appeared, bare breasted, waist-deep in water. Santiago saw her and stood up also, his eyes looking up at the sky, his hands in front of his body, covering his manhood, in the pose of Adam.

"Come swim with me!" Rosa beckoned."

Santiago lowered his gaze for a moment. His eyes drank in Rosa's brown body glazed with river water, her inviting eyes, her smile. He started to say something, but then dove into the current. Swimming underwater, downstream, he could hear only the sound of his heartbeat.

In Acatlan, as in many Mexican towns, the church presides over the town square. Thus it is natural that here, on Sundays after church, the villagers congregate. After the church bells have stopped ringing, the blind old man plays his guitar, families promenade, and the young people engage in an age-old courtship ritual—young women strolling counterclockwise around the square, and young men strolling in the opposite direction.

If you are a young man, and as you stroll, a young woman should give you one violet, this is normal. It is an act of friendship.

If, another time you stroll past each other, and she gives you a second violet, this means that she likes you. It is more than just friendship.

A young man can know a woman many months or even years, and he may, on any given Sunday receive only two violets from her.

If you should stroll past her yet again, and she gives you a third violet, it means she wants to go walking with you.

With all its smiles and glances and feigned disinterest and silent flirtations and flowers—Santiago became fond of this ritual. He didn't need to say anything, only to move—as if through air—nonchalantly.

And it was because of the ritual, after Rosa gave him his third violet, that he took his first walk alone with her. They ambled down through the town, through the orchards, and Rosa led him along a path that wound through the greenery along the riverbanks to a deep pool with large boulders half-submerged in the water. Because it was far away from where the villagers usually swam, it was a private place.

It became their daily habit to walk there. At first Rosa would laugh and joke as they walked along, but soon she learned simply to walk in silence, beside Santiago, taking in the birdsongs, the sounds of the insects and sensing the movements of Santiago's moving, as they walked hand-in-hand.

And so, silently they would arrive at the pool, disrobe, dive into the cool waters and then stretch out on the boulders to bask in the sun.

The night before Santiago was to leave Acatlan, Rosa organized a party in his honor. Because Santiago didn't drink, Enrique's mother served him Turkish coffee in little white cups. All the girls and boys from the village had come, and when the needle was placed on the first record, Santiago took Rosa's hand and led her to the space that had been cleared for dancing. The young men leaned lustily into the steps, and the liquid limbs of the young maidens began to swim under their skirts, their necks curved like the necks of cellos.

In his home town everyone agreed that Santiago, even from a young age, was one of the best dancers, and with his good looks, every time he took to the dance floor, women seemed to float and blossom in his arms, like so many flowers. And so it was that Santiago's mother had begun to chide him—calling him *chupamirto*—hummingbird—and Santiago would tease her back—saying—"Maybe I am the flower—and they are the hummingbirds."

And on this night, it was no different than at home. Protected by the music, Santiago was able to reign in complete silence, taking each girl into his world, guiding each using only the touch of his hand, the inflection of his torso—the insinuations of his eyes.

Santiago's train was scheduled to leave in only one hour. He was sitting with Enrique at a breakfast of *huevos rancheros* with papaya and cold hibiscus tea when Rosa came into the kitchen.

"Would you like to come to the station with us?" asked Enrique.

Rosa smiled, paused for a moment, and then said to Santiago: "When you see what is in your bed, maybe you will not want to leave." She then quickly disappeared.

Santiago looked at Enrique. Enrique shrugged his shoulders. Santiago then got out of his chair and walked up the stairs to the guest room. The door of the guest room was closed.

Santiago placed his hand on the knob and turned it. He pushed the door open. There, on his bed, awaited dozens of calla lilies—one from each girl at the party.

Santiago did not take the train home that day. He stayed on—and each day he and Rosa continued to walk—silently—to the secret pool in the river, where they would disrobe, cool off in the waters, and then bask silently in the sun.

One day, as Rosa was half-slumbering on a boulder beside Santiago, she was awakened by a sudden whirring. A banana tree grew over the pool, and a hummingbird was hovering and sipping just above them. Also drawn to the flower, a wasp was trying to drive off the hummingbird. But the hummingbird was more agile, dancing around the aggressor as it sipped from the flower.

Santiago and Rosa watched until the bird had drunk its fill. Then, suddenly, as if the sky had opened and began to rain, Santiago began to speak.

He began telling her a story about his mother—about when he and his brothers had visited her—after his grandfather's death. He said he had been sitting with his brothers, talking with his mother, when she had excused herself and gone into her bedroom. From where they were sitting, they could hear her putting on a record. They heard the needle touch the plastic and make that scratching sound before the music begins. It was—Santiago said—one of their mother's favorite songs: "Lisbon Antigua," In Old Lisbon.

Santiago said that his mother then began singing to the music. It was extraordinary—he emphasized. It was—he said—the first time they had ever heard her sing.

There was a pause.

Rosa could hear her heart beating wildly, but she tried to remain calm. "How…how does the song go?" She stammered.

There was another pause. Then, softly, Santiago began singing the lyrics.

Rosa did not say a word. She did not breathe. She remained utterly still.

Although Santiago's heart was beginning to open up and lose his fantasy of living a life of silence with his love, as Santiago and Rosa continued their relationship, it was not long before they began to notice that they kept getting on each other's nerves. Because of Rosa's clinging, affectionate, extroverted behavior, Santiago felt as if he were going to be smothered. Therefore, the closer she wanted to get to him, the more he backed away. He had hesitated before moving into the same house, because that would make him dependent on her—or at least interdependent—and he valued a cat-like independence above all things.

If Rosa wanted to be with Santiago all the time, even on weekends, and felt jealous if he went out alone, or with his friends, he felt that he needed more and more space. If Rosa responded to this by continuing to seek maximum contact, his indifference toward her grew even further. He began to take her for granted. Yet, secretly, as much as he felt smothered by her displays of love, he also craved love and felt entitled to it for his fulfillment.

Whenever Christmas or his birthday rolled around, Rosa would lavish upon Santiago the most expensive presents: nice sweaters or tickets for two to Bermuda or Jamaica. He had trouble accepting the presents gracefully, as he did not want to feel obligated to Rosa.

Yet, if Rosa would set eyes on another man, Santiago would show absolutely no tolerance for her disloyalty. Nor, as a business major, did he tolerate her inadequate knowledge of money.

Keeping his distance emotionally allowed him to be in control and to make the big decisions, yet, secretly he craved to relinquish all control. As a lover, his pattern was to seduce physically, but withhold emotionally. He would avoid or minimize both his own feelings and those of Rosa, dismissing emotions with twists of irony. This of course, led to more and more sex, as Rosa attempted to get to the core of him through the one channel—the physical one—he allowed her.

Rosa, on the other hand, suffered from a fear of independence—or even adulthood. She felt herself clinging to him and pursuing him—but she could not resist her natural desire for maximum contact, and had trouble letting go.

In order to try and understand him, Rosa would listen attentively, becoming overly enmeshed in his stories and fleeting displays of real emotion. She found herself acting as a caretaker, catering to Santiago's every whim, while neglecting herself.

She felt she had no right to complain or register her feelings with him if she felt neglected or abused. Thus, she found herself simply trying to cope with anything he dished out—always agreeing to eat at the restaurants he liked, to see the films he wanted to attend and to accept the way he wanted to spend his time on weekends. Because she kept giving more and more—yet receiving less and less—Rosa felt herself developing an actual addiction to her unfulfilling behavior with him. She kept looking for reassurances that he loved her, and that he was not going to abandon her.

If she found Santiago's coolness abusive, she rationalized it—making excuses for him, while burying her own feelings, protecting him from seeing her real self.

Because of the ongoing tensions in their relationship, which each felt both bodily and mentally—they became addicted to passionate, conventional sex—with orgasm—to gain a fleeting sense of unity and a momentary escape from their loneliness and emotional distance.

Lovers are sexually what they are emotionally. It is your pattern of relationship—emotionally—that structures your love life. It is quite possible for you to practice Polynesian lovemaking—but remain caught up emotionally in infant and adolescent levels of emotional adaptation. For instance, your heart may be governed by abandonment and engulfment feelings—stemming from your early childhood—that absolutely shape the emotionally reactive patterns through which you relate to your lover.

Santiago carries in his heart a fear of dependency. He fears that he will be engulfed by his lover. Rosa, on the other hand, fears abandonment and independence—in a sense she fears being an adult. She nourishes a nostalgia for maternal nurturing. Because their opposite fears stimulate each other—they become addicted to each other in order to experience those fears—which do not actually have their source in the relationship, but in their early childhood experiences.

But because neither Santiago nor Rosa realizes this—they both merely act out those fears in the ongoing drama of their relationship—using passionate conventional sex and orgasm as a vacation from themselves.

Because Rosa feels hurt by Santiago's emotional distance, and Santiago fears engulfment by Rosa's fawning attitude, neither of them really feels a connection to the deepest recesses of their heart when they are making love.

If they should attempt to enjoy Polynesian lovemaking together, it would be difficult—as neither she nor Santiago always feels overflowing love for the other.

Yet, the sexual communion felt by sensitive lovers during Polynesian lovemaking is not really a matter of control, as advocated by Taoists and others. It is a matter of both partners yielding the fullness of the sexual-emotional function—surrendering their body, mind, and ego—to an infinity of bliss.

What Santiago and Rosa must do is compassionately and mutually share with each other their own emotional patterns. If they wish to grow beyond the fears that rule their behavior and that structure the ongoing drama of their relationship, they must form a commitment to a bond—a sensitivity to mutually fulfilling behavior. They must both stop dramatizing and acting out the fears deep in their hearts.

After all, an adult cannot be abandoned. She is not going to die, like an infant deprived of her mother's breast. She may only feel that way if she does not get enough reassurance of love. And no adult can be engulfed and smothered.

What Santiago and Rosa must learn to do is to both work on their own fears and have compassion for their partner's fears. Actually, they have chosen each other because they stimulate these fears that have been long hidden in the deep interior landscape of their hearts.

Instead of blaming Santiago for his distance toward her, she could take the very scary step of acknowledging both to herself and to Santiago her deep fears. So she needs first of all just to become honest with herself and with Santiago. She could say something as simple as: "When you go out with your friends every Wednesday night and come home late—and when you act coolly toward me—I feel threatened and abandoned. I need a lot of assurances from you that you love me—either in words or in small gestures that let me know you care. That is how I am built. From my side, I will try to not act on my fears or dramatize my fears by blaming you. I will try to let you get just an inch further away—each day—and notice that I survive—that I am doing OK—and that I am not abandoned."

And Santiago could be honest with Rosa also; he could have compassion both for his fears and for hers. First, if she opens up to him and tells him of her fears, he could acknowledge that he has heard her and takes her seriously (and she could do the same for him). He might say something such as: "I like you, obviously, or I wouldn't be having sex with you. But I feel uncomfortable with a lot of physical contact and closeness and mushiness unless we are having sex. That is how I am. I feel I will be engulfed by your affection and intimacy, and it is scary. But I will attempt not to act on my fears. I realize they are from my childhood, from the distant past—and that I am merely dramatizing them in our relationship. And I will not act on them or dramatize them, but try to let us get just an inch closer every day, and notice that by doing so I have not become drowned or engulfed by you."

If you can tell your partner of your fears, then you will feel good about yourself—you will feel good that you have stood up for your own heart—which is actually the center of your life. And you will learn if your partner really accepts you or not. You will learn if he or she is truly committed to the relationship.

If Rosa fears being abandoned by her lover, then simply by hanging loose and letting Santiago get a little more distant will reinforce her own ability to feel independent. If on the other hand Santiago fears that intimacy is going to engulf him and take something away from him—then he might try giving himself more fully to the relationship—giving in to intimacy—and noticing that he not only survives, but feels great.

If you share your emotional patterns with your lover in this way—then true intimacy and real insight into your relationship develops as a by-product of the conversation. And in such conversations, try to mirror, or repeat, what your partner says, so that your partner really feels that he or she has been listened to caringly. Your relationship then has the chance to become profoundly unified on the level of the heart. When both you and your lover have made such a mutual confession and surrendered—in your hearts—to the relationship, then you do not feel so separate from one another. And you therefore do not seek to overcome a feeling of emotional and physical separation by exploiting the ability of your body and mind to quickly produce orgasm and expel the essence of the life force from your body. Such conventional sexuality is just a dramatization of the feeling of separateness—which is only momentarily mended by sex and orgasm.

Rather—feeling a sense of union—you will cherish the occasion of intimacy as an opportunity to contemplate the flow of life energy—to relax into that current of energy to the point of infinity. Thus, the pleasure of sexual play is raised from its localization and isolation in the genitals to pervade the entire body, mind and heart—infinitely. Over time, your sexual play and everyday lives become more and more about intimacy and relational love.

You can see, then, that when you reach this level in your hearts, control is not needed in order to avoid orgasm. It is a subtle consideration, and demands that you do philosophy not only with your minds—but with your emotional patterns and your bodies.

If Santiago and Rosa should practice meditation and yoga

together, they will begin to notice that in their embrace their energy enjoys flowing upward and inward towards the heart—quite naturally. The benefit is a more fulfilling sense of relationship—not only between themselves, but with everything.

They will have transcended the sexual-emotional orientation of most couples, who, only when they kiss and hug, feel an opportunity to experience a sense of the flow of their life energy moving within themselves. Such couples, in the embrace of conventional sex, find that it provides perhaps the only occasion where they feel they go beyond themselves. Thus, kissing and hugging become a very big deal for them. If they do not have it, they feel isolated, alone and tense.

As Rosa and Santiago share with each other their fears and engage in Polynesian lovemaking from the level of the heart, they will be able to experience profound flows of energy within themselves, and as they persist in the practice of meditation, they will begin to have the experience of feeling that while doing almost anything: eating, going to sleep, waking up, greeting each other, playing with a puppy—they feel profound peace and connectedness. Thus, sexual play will no longer provide their only avenue to feel a sense of relatedness with life energy. They will be able to sit "alone" on a desolate mountain peak and feel utterly in union with Nature. They will know that having that ability is the basis of having a fulfilling relationship.

Once they enter into emotional intimacy they will begin to have the experience that even the love play of their bodies is governed by subtle, but powerful fields of energy that are not confined to the boundaries of their bodies.

In doing so, if Rosa and Santiago watch their own minds—they will see how much their mental images of each other had pervaded their relationship.

After some time together, lovers tend to build up entire image banks about each other. Santiago may have the image that Rosa is a dependent puppy dog, and Rosa may see in her mind a Santiago who is a cool, independent cat. When this happens, it is two image banks relating to each other, rather than two people seeing each other clearly in every moment. But if they ask themselves: What would our love be like if it were free of images—if we could get beyond the fears that define our pattern of relationship?—then they can begin to enjoy a relationship that is radically different.

After all, there is a great difference between the subjective and separative act of entertaining an image in your mind and the relational act of entering into intimate, heartfelt, sensuous, whole-body contact with your lover. The Polynesians, who were very natural and positive about their bodies, feelings and sex enjoyed a sexuality that was essentially imageless, and they used to laugh at the early European explorers, whose minds were fixated on images of various body parts.

If your mind is free of thought—as it will be if you and your lover share with each other your fears and meditate together—then you will feel a deep sense of union with everything, and of peace. In that state of mind, you can really contemplate the flow of energy between you and your lover. Sexuality—in such a state—is not about finding a sense of release from bodily, emotional or mental tension. It is not a dramatization of overcoming a sense of separateness, drama and doubt. It is not about throwing off your energy through the spasm of orgasm.

Sexual play becomes transformed. When embracing your love, you are able to enter into the flow of energy until it becomes radiant, to the level of infinity. In that state, there is no duality, and you can play and relax in such a heavenly embrace for hours. Your intimacy is about the embrace itself, not the conventional result of embracing. It is not about release. It is about fullness.

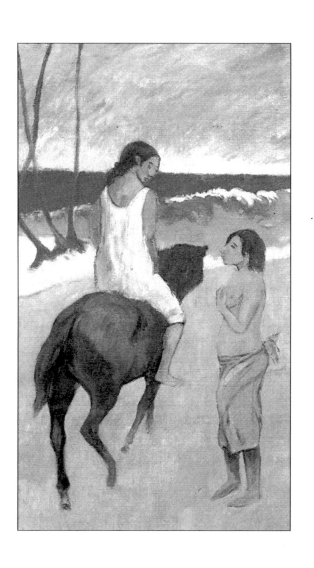

Weaving Together

*D*o you and your lover measure the success of your relation-ship by the power and frequency of your orgasms? Then consider this: Orgasms—like a lot of things—have two sides. In fact, Marquesian islanders have two expressions for orgasm. *Manini* (literally "sweet") refers to the feelings of pleasure, release and well-being that follow this form of sexual expression. On the other hand, the words *ua pe nei au* are used by a man to convey to his lover that he has ejaculated. They mean, "I am rotten." The expression is thus something like the French metaphor for orgasm: "the small death."

When you feel that more and better orgasms will create a bond that will never die between you and your lover—you are thinking about the sweet, *manini* feelings orgasm can produce. However, as more and more couples become more adept at conventional sex, and thus have more and more orgasms, divorce rates and the problems of sexless marriages keep increasing. The problem with "the small death" of orgasm is that the feeling behind the second expression—"I am rotten"—can ruin a relationship rather than strengthen it.

Such feelings arise because conventional orgasm is part of a cycle that is chemically addictive. Through millions of years of evolution our brains have been chemically programmed to crave behavior important to our survival. An example is our craving for fat. To almost everyone, a potato with a big pat of butter and a spoonful of sour cream is more appetizing than a potato with just salt and pepper. We feel this way because for millions of years—as our species fought to survive—fat was not always available. But our bodies need fat. Therefore—over time—the primitive parts of our brain became programmed to make us want to eat all the fat we can every time we encounter some. One reason many people are obese is that they actually eat the amount of fat that the primitive part of their brain makes them crave.

When you are actually devouring an order of French fries or a bag of potato chips, your brain is releasing a chemical called dopamine. Dopamine makes you crave things. It makes you feel you cannot do without them. If you eat almost any high-calorie food—the primitive part of your brain rewards you by shooting you with a big blast of dopamine. It is dopamine that tells you to go for the cream puff or the ice cream rather than the broccoli. Even though you may be in a supermarket, surrounded with thousands of times more food than you can eat—your primitive brain can only think: "Eat a LOT of calories NOW—if you want to survive."

When we were cave men and did not have a refrigerator full of ice cream, butter and sour cream—our craving for fat helped us survive. If we killed a deer, we gorged ourselves on fat. And that big helping of fat carried us over until the next time we could get some. However, now when we are surrounded by fats the craving no longer contributes to our survival; we simply end up eating too many of them. Craving now contributes—instead—to obesity and heart disease. Dopamine is the addiction drug.

In the same way that eating a lot of fat at one sitting once helped us survive, having sex with a variety of sexual partners was also—at one time—an evolutionary activity, because it allowed the most genetic diversity. The more genetically diverse a species is, the better it can adapt to a changing environment. Having an orgasm—especially with an attractive new partner—gives you the most massive blast of dopamine possible. However, once this takes place, your brain no longer needs the high level of dopamine. The neurochemical has accomplished its mission: It has produced in you the behavior that has the most probability of creating another, genetically diverse, human being. You have just broadcasted your DNA to another new partner. What goes up, must come down. After reaching peak levels during orgasm—dopamine levels start to drop off sharply.

After orgasm, Nature begins flooding your brain with another chemical—prolactin. Prolactin helps you shut down dopamine production. It also makes you disinterested in sex. In men this disinterest takes place almost immediately after orgasm. Men want to roll over and go to sleep. In women the dopamine-induced disinterest can take many days.

However, as prolactin levels rise, they can cause not only disinterest in sex, but anxiety, headaches, depression, menstrual problems and feelings of anger and irritability. If you experience these feelings you may start over-eating, or compulsively play video games in order to pump up your domanine levels again.

Most likely, you will not attribute these negative feelings to sex—after all—you have been taught to believe that conventional sex that includes orgasm creates lasting harmony and love. Thus, you might begin to project these negative prolactin-induced feelings onto your partner. Suddenly you might see your partner's faults. You might notice that your partner may not look as attractive as before. However, if you should see—out of the corner of your eye—a hot-looking stranger walking down the street—you might suddenly feel a craving to run out the door and have hot sex with that stranger. That sudden craving for sex with a stranger is your dopamine kicking in again—telling you that you must have it. And, as already mentioned, if you do go have sex with the sexy new thing—you are engaging in evolutionary behavior—genetic diversity. The more partners you have, the more you broadcast your DNA, the more genetically diverse your offspring will be, and that increases the chances of survival of the species.

Conventional sex and orgasm, then, are programmed by your brain to be a chemically addictive cycle. Your body, life and emotions are—to an extent—puppets of the dopamine/prolactin cycle. If you are addicted to conventional sex you must suffer through the chemical highs and lows that form that addictive cycle. Your body and mind know subconsciously that after orgasm there is going to be a period of time when your prolactin levels are high and irritability and depression are going to set in. To avoid this sudden plummeting of dopamine levels—if you are sexually addicted—you might resort to almost any means to stimulate yourself to achieve another orgasm and get another dopamine rush. However, this may just devitalize you even further, forming an endless cycle.

So, having wonderful sex can actually lead to relationship conflict a week after orgasm—as dopamine levels fall. Yet, if you are like most couples who engage in conventional sex, you remain on a chemical roller-coaster of dopamine highs and prolactin lows. In your low periods, you will tend to begin to view your lover in a negative light and develop a craving for someone new.

But what if you can actually orchestrate your neurochemicals so that they are not addictive? By enjoying Polynesian lovemaking, you can actually bypass the entire cycle of dopamine/prolactin addiction. This is because Polynesian lovemaking allows you to flood yourself with another chemical—oxytocin. Whereas dopamine is the "Lust" chemical, oxytocin has been called the "Cuddling" chemical, the "Caring" chemical, the "Bonding" chemical and the "Love" chemical. Oxytocin increases when you really love someone, when you have a pet you care deeply for and when you dive deep into the heart during meditation or Polynesian-style love.

Oxytocin makes you feel like lavishing nurturing affection on your partner—giving your partner a massage, listening to your partner's feelings—touching your lover with real affection rather than just grabbing or stimulating. As you do these things, your oxytocin levels will increase, and so will your partner's. Oxytocin is the hormone that is at high levels when you have an open heart. It also is a chemical that makes you live longer, healthier and enjoy a more glowing life.

When you fall in love, your oxytocin levels are high. Because the chemical is associated with heartfelt love, it makes your lover look more and more attractive, even with all his or her faults, than any stranger possibly could.

If you enjoy Polynesian lovemaking you can actually create so much oxytocin that it will help you form a strong—heartfelt bond with your love. And because your loving has blossomed into a more heartfelt mode—you will not be so tempted to get caught up in the excessive highs and lows of addictive conventional sex with orgasm. After sex, you will not be engaging in addictive behavior to pump up your dopamine levels. You will not be looking around for exciting sexual partners while in the throes of a prolactin-induced negativity.

Playboy rats, when injected with oxytocin, actually stop playing around and began preferring sex with the same partner. Oxytocin is the "I've grown accustomed to your face" drug. It makes your lover— however plain—look more loveable than anyone else. And it makes you feel like loving with genuine affection—not just lust.

Oxytocin reduces cravings and addictions. Drug-addicted rats injected with oxytocin lose interested in heroin, cocaine and morphine. By exploring Polynesian lovemaking, you are actually healing yourself and your lover of addictive behavior in general. You are creating a new neurochemistry. Because oxytocin increases sexual sensitivity at the same time that it decreases cravings, Polynesian lovemaking without conventional orgasm can be completely satisfying.

Whereas the dopamine/prolactin cycle leads to promiscuous and addictive behavior—oxytocin supports a peaceful mind and heart, and monogamy.

For sensitive lovers, the big "O" is not found in orgasm—but in any behavior that enhances production of the love chemical, oxytocin.

Your life is like a blank canvas. You can paint it any way you like. It is up to you. To increase your level of oxytocin and live in deepening intimacy with your beloved—tend toward the following behaviors:

1. Take very good care of yourself. Pamper yourself. Every fulfilling relationship is based on giving. However, you can give to your partner only what you have. If you are full of stress, tension and stagnant, blocked energy, that is all you will able to give to your partner. If you are full of bliss and vibrancy, that is what you will have available to share. So, if you want to make love soul-to-soul, not just genitals-to-genitals, first learn to meditate, get a

massage often so that your areas of blocked energy are dissolved and your body feels full of vitality and sweet energy, discover how it feels to circulate your energy by learning Tai C'hi or yoga. Practice daily. Get plenty of rest. Then, when you feel your body is full of delicious swirling energy, when you feel like singing the body electric, when you embrace a tree and can feel deeply into its heart, you really have something precious and sacred to share with your beloved.

2. Make love only with another soul who has learned to dive deeply within his or her own heart in meditation, who takes care of his or her own body and emotions, who has a sense of inner silence and bliss. If you have been taking good care of yourself, you will be able to sense the qualities of and to attract such an open, loving partner.

3. Share energy with your partner. Meditate together daily. Do yoga or Tai C'hi together. Explore giving full-body massage to each other, massaging not only the physical body, but also becoming sensitive to the fabric of subtle energy that is being woven together between your two increasingly relaxed and sensitive bodies. Discover how it feels to simply embrace your partner after massage, without having sex. Become sensitive to the energies you begin to feel flowing between you in such an embrace.

4. Begin to explore Polynesian lovemaking very gradually with your partner. Genuine change develops slowly. As you both become more relaxed, you will be weaving together deeper and deeper levels of energy and love.

5. Learn to weave together your sexual and spiritual energies: When in a sexual embrace with your partner, slowly weave together your energies by moving more and more slowly, keeping aware of your breath and of the flows of energy between you. Resist the urge to move faster and faster. If you feel the urge to focus on more stimulation and to tense your body around it, do just the opposite. Simply stop moving. Stop, and just radiate to each other the fullness of light you feel within your hearts. Simply embrace and rest together within this light. Then weave this light back into your sexual energy by beginning to move again, slowly, but only enough to keep the male erect and the female interested. From time to time, shift into another comfortable, relaxing position and continue weaving together, always sensing the circulation of energies.

6. Whatever emotions or fantasies arise during lovemaking, just allow them to come into your mind—then let them go.

After making love in this way, separate slowly, gently. Even though you may have made love for hours, you will not feel exhausted. You will not feel as if you want to roll over and go to sleep. You will not feel "I am rotten." You will feel full of energy. You will still feel sexually interested and interesting. You will feel alive.

When you begin to explore Polynesian lovemaking with your partner, do so gradually and without imposing any sense of obligation. Just play with Polynesian passion and find out what it feels like. Do not force it on yourself or on your partner. If you feel like making love in your old, conventional manner, full of passion and leading to orgasm, go ahead. At other times, combine conventional sex with Polynesian loving. This will bring more and more awareness to your periods of physical intimacy. You will begin to experience how your desire and your spirit interact within you. In that growing awareness you will realize that so-called Polynesian lovemaking has little at all to do with your many images of a place called Polynesia: It is, instead, about weaving the strands of your life into a peaceful place in the heart that is beyond space, time and images.

I'll see you there.

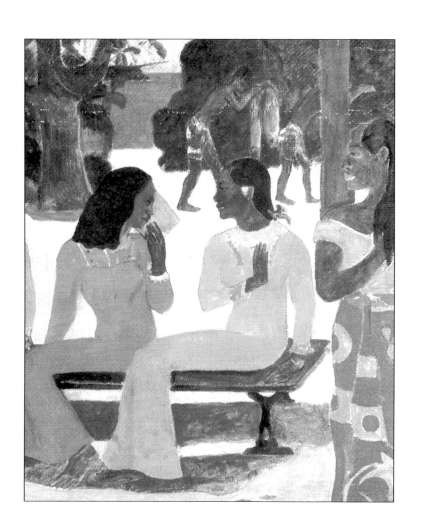

Polynesian Passion: Your Experience

*T*he next book on Polynesian lovemaking will be written by the readers of this book. It will be composed mostly of the experiences of couples who have taken the time and care to explore the hidden depths of Polynesian lovemaking. Ideally, I would like to hear from every couple who has read this book, and to hear in detail what your experiences were like emotionally, physically, and in terms of the effect on your relationship.

If your response is published in my next book, your names, of course, will not be used and your e-mail address will be confidential. Please visit my website, **PolynesianLove.com** and click on "Experiences" to submit your responses. Also check the website to find out about workshops and new Polynesian lovemaking information.

If you wish receive newsletters and information about my "Still Sensing" workshops, please sign up by sending an e-mail to: **news@PolynesianLove.com**.

In case you have some difficulties thinking of a way to tell us about your experiences—the following questions may help you get started:

1. Have you and/or your lover practiced meditation: going to the calm space between the breaths?
2. Do you practice meditation daily?
3. What is your experience in meditation?

4. Do you practice meditation together before you begin making love?

5. Have you and your lover explored Polynesian lovemaking?

6. If so, what was your experience like?

7. What about your bodily sensations?

8. Did you feel an accumulation of energy in the genital area?

9. Did it make you feel like simply surrendering to the pleasure of a genital orgasm?

10. Did you find yourself seeking release through genital stimulation, or did you feel some element of energy—emotion in the heart?

11. Was the act of sex you engaged in a loveless, manipulative game, to secure your own orgasm—or did you really feel something for your partner; did you feel as if you are really sharing vital and emotional energy with your partner?

12. Were you increasing stimulation, increasing bodily movements in order to increase the intensity of sensations?

13. Did you feel addicted to orgasm?

14. Did you find yourself or your partner trying to achieve orgasm even though you want to explore the process of Polynesian lovemaking?

15. Can you make love for a prolonged period, but feel unsatisfied unless there is an orgasm?

16. Do you feel you partner wants you to have an orgasm or at least to fake an orgasm, or to bring him or her to orgasm?

17. What happens when you stop going towards orgasm, when you stop all bodily movements and allow your breath to take its own form?

18. Does it become long and deep naturally?

19. And what becomes of the accumulation of sensation in the genital area when you breathe deeply?

20. Does it dissolve and circulate throughout the whole body?

21. Do you depend almost exclusively on sexual intercourse to feel energy moving within your body, or are there other occasions when you feel really connected to an intense flow of energy, for instance, meditation, Tai C'hi, and so on?

22. Do you really feel cut off from blissfulness in your life except in those moments of deep passion during sex?

23. Is it possible for you to feel that same intensity of pleasure in other activities, or in all conditions?

24. Do you feel anything in the region of your heart?

25. What if you cease all movement, allow your breathing to become natural, and hold your lover close against yourself—heart-to-heart?

26. Do you feel a radiance or light pulsing from the region of the heart?

27. When you are in a sexual embrace with your partner, do you feel love, or just the stimulation of desire?

28. Do you feel intense emotion for your lover, and do you express this fully by submitting bodily and sensitively to your lover?

29. Or are you preoccupied with mental phenomenon?

30. Is your mind filled with sexual images?

31. Do you imagine, for instance, being with someone else?

32. Is your mind filled with sexual fantasies, not really conscious of what is happening physically, in the present, with your lover—here and now?

33. Are you really experiencing the body, or just the mind?

34. Are you using fantasy to motivate the body?

35. Or are you surrendered to an imageless, thought-free, fully relational and radiant flow of energy and sensation between your partner and yourself?

36. Do you find yourself imagining a situation of conflict—such as rape, in order to stimulate genital orgasm?

37. Do you find that you are trying to avoid showing signs of obvious passion, or to withdraw your attention from physical sensations by imagining things that have no erotic content?

38. If so, is it possible for you to simply observe this and bring attention back to your lover?

39. Is your energy localized in the area of the genitals—or do you feel full-body radiance? Can you contemplate the circulation of energy within your entire body/mind?

40. Are you using your attention to exploit the sexual function, or are you sacrificing the entire apparatus of attention to pure radiance?

41. Are you trying to avoid orgasm, in order to "be spiritual" through a process that is primarily mechanical?

42. Or are you transcending orgasm through love, through sensitive attention to your lover and through radiance at the level of the heart?

43. Have you experienced an orgasm?

44. If so, did you use it to relieve mental, emotional and physical tension?

45. Do you still feel desire for your partner or do you now feel like being separate from him or her?

46. Do you both tend to have or want orgasm when you are exploring Polynesian lovemaking?

47. Did you follow the guidelines closely or loosely?

48. How about communication and emotions between you and your lover—have those improved?

49. Do you feel you understand how to explore Polynesian lovemaking?

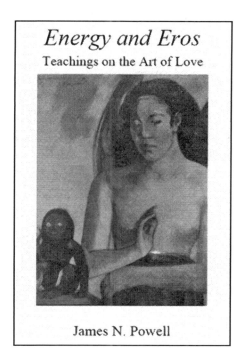

Energy and Eros
Teachings on the Art of Love

James N. Powell

Teachings of sacred sexuality from traditional Polynesia, Taoist China and Tantric India. Originally published by William Morrow in the United States, it was subsequently translated in Spain and Japan (Hosei University Press). It was in Japan that the book sparked a slow-love sexual revolution that is now spreading worldwide.

- Learn the way of Tantra as practiced in ancient India
- Learn the Tao of love as practiced in ancient China
- Learn the way of Polynesian love as practiced in ancient Polynesia
- Learn the way of loving that Japanese women are asking their boyfriends and husbands to try

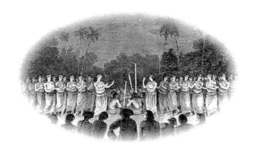

**Also by
James Powell**

Energy and Eros

The Tao of Symbols

Derrida for Beginners

Deconstruction for Beginners

Postmodernism for Beginners

Eastern Philosophy for Beginners

Mandalas: The Dynamics
of Vedic Symbolism